November,
2001.

**Earl Mindell, R.Ph., Ph.D.,
is also the author of**

....

Earl Mindell's Supplement Bible

Earl Mindell's Secret Remedies

Earl Mindell's Anti-Aging Bible

Earl Mindell's Soy Miracle Cookbook

Earl Mindell's Soy Miracle

Earl Mindell's Food as Medicine

Earl Mindell's Vitamin Bible

Earl Mindell's
New Herb Bible

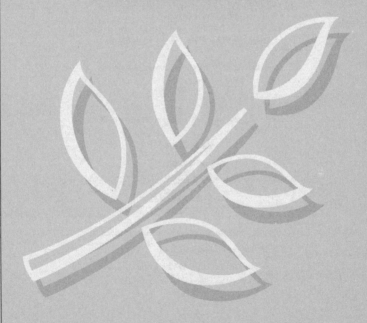

Earl Mindell, R.Ph., Ph.D.

A Fireside Book • *Published by Simon & Schuster*

FIRESIDE
Rockefeller Center
1230 Avenue of the Americas
New York, NY 10020

Designed by Barbara M. Bachman

Manufactured in the United States of America

1 3 5 7 9 10 8 6 4 2

Library of Congress Cataloging-in-Publication Data

Mindell, Earl.
[New herb bible]
Earl Mindell's new herb bible / Earl Mindell. — [Completely rev.
and updated ed.]
p.   cm.
Includes bibliographical references and index.
1. Herbs—Therapeutic use.   I. Title.
RM666.H33M562   2000
615'.321—dc21   99-43320
CIP

ISBN 0-684-85639-5

This book is dedicated to Gail, Alannah, Evan,

my parents and family, my friends and associates,

and to the continuing happiness and health

of people everywhere.

Acknowledgments

I wish to express my deep and lasting appreciation to my friends and associates, who have assisted me in the preparation of this book, especially: J. Kenney, Ph.D.; Linus Pauling, Ph.D.; Harold Segal, Ph.D.; Bernard Bubman, R.Ph.; Mel Rich, R.Ph.; Sal Messineo, Pharm.D., R.Ph.; Arnold Fox, M.D.; Dennis Huddleson, M.D.; Stewart Fisher, M.D.; the late Robert Mendelsohn, M.D.; Gershon Lesser, M.D.; David Velkoff, M.D.; Rory Jaffee, M.D.; Vicki Hufnagel, M.D.; Donald Cruden, O.D.; Joel Strom, D.D.S.; Nathan Sperling, D.D.S. A special thanks to Rob McCaleb of the Herb Research Foundation for his assistance. I would also like to thank Carol Colman Gerber and my editor, Caroline Sutton, for their help with this project. A special thanks to my agent, Richard Curtis, for his support throughout the years. Finally, I would like to express my gratitude to Dominion Herbal College, where I received my degrees as a chartered herbalist and as a master herbalist.

Contents

Before You Begin this Book

Ten years ago, when I first told a friend that I was writing a book on herbs, he looked startled and said, "Why, Earl, I had no idea that you could cook!"

Today, his comment seems laughable but, back then, most people still thought that herbs were only something you added to tomato sauce or sprinkled on a salad.

What a difference a decade makes!

According to a recent survey, one-third of all Americans today use herbal supplements and related products. Once relegated to a small shelf in the back of the store, herbs now account for about 25 percent of all sales in natural food stores. There are now row upon row of herbal supplements not just where you'd expect to find them—in natural food stores—but also in conventional pharmacies, discount stores, supermarkets, and even in doctors' offices. Aspirin and acetaminophen now stand side by side with herbs such as echinacea, goldenseal, kava, valerian, ginseng, and St. John's wort. If, as the saying goes, money talks, Americans are loudly voicing their support for herbal products. In 1994, Americans spent 1.6 billion dollars on herbal preparations; by 1998, that number had nearly tripled, to $4 billion in retail sales. I predict that the market will continue to grow exponentially.

Sales of herbal products have skyrocketed since Congress passed the 1994 Dietary Supplement Health and Education Act (DSHEA), which radically changed the way supplements can be sold and marketed in the United States. The law lifted decades of regulatory barriers that had made it difficult, if not impossible, to bring new supplements to market. The law also made it easier for manufacturers to make health claims for their products as long as they had scientific backing. If an herb was a proven treatment for cold or headache, the manufacturer could say so on the label. This made it easier than ever for people to find and use the appropriate herbal products.

The herbal revolution has done nothing less than change the way medicine is being practiced. Once dismissed as quackery, traditional remedies are now getting a close look from mainstream scientists. The United States Congress has established the office of Alternative Medicine under the National Institutes of Health to study alternative medicine, including herbs. Recently, an entire issue of the conservative *Journal of the American Medical Association* was devoted to exploring various forms of alternative medicine. So much has happened since the *Herb Bible* was published in 1992, that it has become necessary to update this book. Not only do I introduce scores of new herbs in this new edition, but I also include the latest scientific findings on herbs that were listed in the old edition. Similar to the old *Herb Bible,* the new *Herb Bible* is designed so that it can be used by both the novice and the experienced herbal consumer.

In a sense, as we embark on a new millennium, we've come full circle. When I was growing up in Canada, my parents often relied on herbs and natural medicine to treat the common illnesses of childhood. However, by the time I started pharmacy school in 1958, the pill-popping era was just dawning. By the time I graduated and entered practice, there seemed to be a pill for whatever ailed us. Have a sore throat? Take an antibiotic. Think a headache is coming on? Reach for an aspirin. Need to drop some weight or pick up some energy? Try amphetamines. Want to calm down? A tranquilizer will help you. This was also the dawn of the space age. The United States was preparing to send a man to the moon in a space capsule. Therefore, it was only logical to believe that we would soon be able to cure the common cold, flu, acne, and various catastrophic illnesses with time-release capsules. The notion that lifestyle, diet, or exercise could possibly influence health was considered unscientific and profoundly silly. "Scientific" remedies were not hard to find, however. They were widely advertised and came packaged in attractive boxes, bottles, or blister packs. Natural remedies—the kind our grandmothers and great-grandmothers relied on—were dismissed as pure hokum. These were the days when there seemed to be nothing that nature could do that humans could not do better.

Against this backdrop, I reluctantly registered for the required course in *pharmacognosy,* the study of drugs derived from plants. My classmates and I disparagingly called the course "weeds and seeds," and thought that it was utterly weird. We went on field trips and foraged for plants known for their medicinal value. With my own hands, I picked them, dried them, and with an old-fashioned mortar and pestle, turned them into useful drugs. In the process, my skepticism about natural remedies began to fade and I started studying the literature some might call the lore of natural remedies. I was astonished to discover that people had been using natural remedies for thousands of years to successfully treat a wide variety of ills, ranging from heartburn to heart disease. In fact, prior to World War II, herbal medications were listed side-by-side with chemical drugs in the U.S. *Pharmacopeia,* the official listing of accepted medicines. Even today, nearly 50 percent of the thousands of drugs commonly used and prescribed are either derived from plant sources or contain chemical imitations of plant compounds. The list is impressive:

- *Digitalis, a potent cardiotonic, is derived from the foxglove plant.*
- *Aspirin is a chemical imitation of salicin, found in the bark of the white willow tree.*
- *Reserpine, a blood pressure medicine, is actually an ancient remedy from India derived from an Asian shrub.*
- *Ephedrine and pseudoephedrine, found in many over-the-counter cold remedies, are derived from the ephedra plant, used in China to treat colds and flu for more than five thousand years!*
- *Quinine, a famous malaria treatment, and quinidine, an antiarrhythmic medication, are made from the bark of the cinchona tree.*
- *Vincristine and vinblastine, two of our most successful cancer treatments, are derived from the rosy periwinkle tree, native to*

*southern Madagascar. Medicine derived from this plant has
saved the lives of thousands of victims of childhood leukemia.*
- *Taxol, derived from the bark of the Pacific Yew tree, has been
used successfully to treat advanced ovarian cancer.*
- *Penicillin, the grandfather of antibiotics, is actually a mold, an
organism produced by a fungus, a primitive plant.*

Thus, I owe my lifelong interest in herbal medicine to the courses I took
in pharmacognosy. After graduation, I began collecting antique herbal
guides, often called *herbals,* some of which are more than two centuries
old. But I never took my herbals to the pharmacy with me, because
herbalism was considered obsolete. Indeed, not long after I graduated,
pharmacognosy was dropped from the list of required courses by many
pharmacy schools. Ironically, many schools have reintroduced the
course and many others are considering it.

The major reason for the decline in herbalism was not the herbs'
inefficacy but economics. Herbs are not as profitable as drugs. In the
United States, most herbs are not recognized as drugs or as having any
medicinal value. Rather, they are classified as food or food additives.
Even if an herb is known to be beneficial as a medicine, it cannot be
sold as a drug until it receives the official stamp of approval by the Food
and Drug Administration, and approval does not come quickly, easily,
or cheaply. Where the introduction of new drugs is concerned, the
United States is one of the most restrictive countries in the world. The
extensive testing required to achieve official drug status, that is, to prove
a substance is safe and effective, can cost hundreds of millions of dollars
and take many years. This explains why the cost of the average prescription has risen tenfold since 1950!

Moreover, natural substances cannot be patented. When a pharmaceutical company creates a new drug, the company is given a twenty-
year exclusive right to market that product, so that the company can
recoup its research and development costs. Were a pharmaceutical
company to simply package an herb, the company would receive no
such market protection. Thus, there is little incentive to spend time and
money investigating the potential benefits of an herb that people can
grow themselves or that competitors are free to market. It's not surprising, therefore, that many pharmaceutical houses have lost interest in

pursuing plant drugs altogether, and instead have focused their research and development efforts on new synthetic medications. An unfortunate consequence of this shift in emphasis to synthetic drugs was that many time-honored natural remedies were displaced and, at least for a while, forgotten.

Today, however, we are witnessing a renewed interest in herbal remedies, not only on the part of alternative physicians but from traditional medical practitioners as well. One reason is the recognition that, although synthetic drugs have certainly performed many miracles and saved countless lives, they have not turned out to be the "silver bullet" that pharmacologists hoped they would be. Virtually all of these drugs have well-known side effects, ranging from the unpleasant to the lethal. In many cases, they are not even effective. For example, antibiotics, for all their ability to defeat bacterial infections, are essentially useless against viruses, and many of the diseases that plague us today, from Shanghai flu to AIDS to chronic fatigue syndrome, are viral syndromes. What's even worse is that, due to the overuse of antibiotics, we are now threatened by new and deadlier strains of antibiotic resistant bacteria. One-third of all strains of streptococcus pneumonia are now resistant to one or more antibiotics. Once easily cured by penicillin, 90 percent of all staph infections are now resistant to this antibiotic, and some new strains are resistant to all drugs.

Another reason for the growing interest in herbal remedies is that we now know that many over-the-counter medications can be hazardous. For example, many consumers turned to acetaminophen as a supposed safe alternative to aspirin, because they feared that aspirin would irritate stomachs or lead to Reye's syndrome in children. Recently, we have learned that acetaminophen combined with excessive alcohol consumption can cause serious liver damage. Antacids, among the most widely used over-the-counter drugs, can actually cause stomach irritation. As every cold or allergy sufferer knows, many popular antihistamines cause drowsiness or excitability, and trigger a rebound effect, resulting in more congestion.

Perhaps the major reason for our renewed interest in herbalism can be attributed to the new emphasis on preventive medicine. The pendulum of science is on its return swing, and we now know that lifestyle and nutrition play significant roles in averting disease. There is a growing recognition that herbs, too, can play a vital role in promoting wellness. Unlike drugs, many herbs are taken as *tonics,* that is, like many vitamins, they can be used primarily to maintain good health. Studies show that there are herbs that can reduce cholesterol, improve circulation, and even prevent cancer. Some herbs have been shown to enhance immune function, thus helping the body to fight disease. Obviously, most of us would prefer to take an herb that would help us stay healthy than a drug when we are sick!

Even as we in the United States were moving away from natural remedies, herbs were being studied and used very successfully abroad. Foreign medical journals are filled with reports of herbs found to be useful in treating cancer, heart disease, and other serious ailments. In countries such as England, Germany, France, China, and Japan, herbs are recognized as valid remedies and are often incorporated in conventional medical treatment. In Germany, herbal medicine is so widely used that there is a separate government entity—Commission E of the Federal Health Agency—that has evaluated the use and efficacy of hundreds of herbs and natural products. As a result, in Germany, a doctor may prescribe the herb valerian for cases of mild anxiety and the patent drug Valium when a stronger drug is needed. Saw palmetto (used to treat enlarged prostate) and St. John's wort (used to treat depression) have been used safely in Germany and other European countries for decades, yet are only just being discovered in the United States. Throughout Europe, herbal remedies and over-the-counter drugs are sold side by side. A British cold sufferer can choose between a packaged herbal cold remedy and a conventional cold capsule.

In natural food stores, herb shops, and even in many drugstores and chain stores around the United States, we now see packaged herbal remedies similar to those that are so popular in Europe. Go into a drugstore or health food store and you are likely to find packages of ginkgo capsules and ginseng extract next to the vitamins and cold medications. However, there is still a great deal of confusion about how to use herbs. Unfortunately, there are few places to go for information. Your local pharmacist probably can't answer your questions because, chances are, he never took a course in pharmacognosy. Most doctors know little about herbs. And the village shaman, the traditional medicine man or woman, has gone the way of the milkman!

Standard herb guides tend to be quite detailed and eclectic, because they are geared to people who have the time and space to grow, dry, and prepare their own remedies, and are able to decode the jargon typical of old-fashioned herbals. My goal in writing the *Herb Bible* is to help close this information gap. Here, I might interject that educating people about alternative approaches to health care is something that I have enjoyed doing for many years. In 1979, I wrote *Earl Mindell's Vitamin Bible,* which has been revised for the twenty-first century and is still widely read today. It is generally regarded as one of the books that helped to popularize vitamin use in the United States. When I first wrote the *Vitamin Bible,* vitamins were viewed as being for health food types only and health food stores were about the only place where you could buy anything more exotic than a standard multivitamin. Today, vitamins are sold everywhere, from the corner drugstore to fashionable department stores, side by side with herbs.

The *Herb Bible* has a mission similar to that of the *Vitamin Bible.* Initially written for the novice, the *New Herb Bible* is written for both the new and experienced user of herbal products. Most of the herbs included in the *Herb Bible* are readily available in most herb shops and health stores, and are also easy to use.

In the first chapter, I explain exactly what herbs are, how they work, and how to buy them. I have assessed hundreds of herbs in use in the United States and have compiled a list called the Hot Hundred. To show how rapidly the herbal landscape has changed, this new edition of the *Herb Bible* contains twenty-eight new Hot Hundred entries, which appear in Chapter 2. These herbs are becoming popular because they are particularly useful for the kinds of ailments that afflict modern men and women. I describe exactly what each herb does and how to use it.

"Traditional Favorites," a selection of time-honored herbal remedies that are still popular today, are reviewed in Chapter 3. In Chapter 4, "Herbs from around the World," you will learn about age-old remedies from China, India, Tibet, South America, and also those used by Native Americans in the United States. "The Herbal Medicine Cabinet," in Chapter 5, will tell you about the herbs that no household should be without. Chapter 6, "A Woman's Body," deals with problems that affect women and explains how herbs can provide significant relief. Chapter 7, "A Man's Body," offers herbal solutions to common problems that afflict men. I have included a major new section in this book, Chapter 8, "Anti-Aging Herbs." In Chapter 9, "Looking Good," I discuss herbal personal grooming products that can be used by both sexes, including the latest in herbal skin care. "Aromatherapy," the increasingly widespread practice of using scented oils for healing, is covered in Chapter 10.

Herbal medicine is not a panacea for all of our ills. There is no substitute for a healthy lifestyle. Prevention is still the best medicine and, in my opinion, always will be. There are times, however, when conventional medicine is absolutely essential. Anyone who has ever been treated successfully with zithromax, who had a strep infection that did not develop into rheumatic fever thanks to amoxicillin, or who beat cancer thanks to chemotherapy owes a debt of gratitude to the pharmaceutical houses that developed these drugs. There should be room, however, for a wide variety of treatment options, and I believe that herbal medicine deserves a place high on that list.

This book does not encourage the self-diagnosis and treatment of disease. If you are seriously ill, you should receive proper medical attention. There are many situations, however, in which it may be appropriate to self-medicate. Few of us call the doctor every time we get a headache, develop a cold, get indigestion, suffer menstrual cramps, or experience the aches and pains of mild arthritis. Most of us rely on over-the-counter medications to treat these relatively benign problems. This book will show you how to select and use natural herbal remedies for these everyday problems. If the condition becomes severe or persists for more than a few days, I feel it is advisable to call your physician.

IMPORTANT:

If you are now taking any drugs, either over-the-counter or prescription, or have any medical conditions or problems, it is wise to consult a naturally oriented physician who is aware of herb/drug interactions and any potentially dangerous side effects *before* taking any herbal remedies.

CHAPTER 1

What Is an Herb?

The word herb has usually been used to refer to any plant or plant part valued for its medicinal, savory, or aromatic qualities. For the purposes of this book, herb means any plant or plant-derived substance that is primarily used for medicinal purposes.

There are approximately 380,000 species of plants on earth that we have identified, and several hundred thousand that have yet to be discovered. Right now, many scientists are desperately trying to catalogue the plants in the Amazon rain forest in the belief that there are thousands of potential plant cures that are rapidly being destroyed by development. Of the number of known plants, about 260,000 are classified as *higher plants,* which means that they contain chlorophyll and perform a process called *photosynthesis.* In photosynthesis, plants utilize the energy provided by sunlight to manufacture carbohydrates from carbon dioxide and water. All the members of the higher plant group have the potential to offer medical benefits. Only 10 percent, however, have actually been studied for this purpose.

In this book, I usually refer to each herb by its two names: the familiar name by which it is commonly known and a Latin botanical name describing its genus and species. The genus or first name is the general grouping of plants by family. Although plants in a given genus are not identical, they have certain similar characteristics. The species is a more specific way of defining each plant's distinctive qualities. For example, onions, garlic, and chives are all members of the *Allium* genus. However, each of these herbs is classified as a different species.

In rare cases, however, I do not include the botanical name for a particular herb. Some herbal products are not derived from the whole plant; rather they are biologically active extracts. A case in point is *bromelain,* an enzyme that is extracted from pineapple that is sold as bromelain, not pineapple. In other cases, an herbal supplement may contain a combination of herbs that are marketed under one name.

■ How Do Herbs Work?

The living cells of plants can be likened to miniature chemical factories. They take in the raw materials carbon dioxide, water, and sunlight, and convert them into useful nutrients. Oxygen is a by-product of this process. Herbs are a rich source of *phytochemicals,* compounds that are pharmacologically active, meaning that they exert a profound effect on certain animal tissues and organs. Therefore, they can be used as drugs in treating, curing, or preventing disease. A plant may consist of several components, including leaves, roots, fruit, flowers, bark, stems, or seeds. Any of these parts may contain the active ingredients that give the plant its medicinal properties.

The herbal pharmacy is a rich one. There are herbs that target specific organ systems, and there are herbs that are used as general tonics to promote overall health. There are herbs that soothe pain and inflammation, and still other herbs that work to reduce muscle spasm. Some herbs have a stimulating effect; others have a relaxing effect. Some kill bacteria; others activate the body's own immune system so that it can ward off invading organisms.

Many herbs contain *antioxidants,* important compounds that protect against potentially dangerous chemicals called *free radicals.* Free radicals are produced in our bodies as a natural byproduct of energy production. If not tightly controlled, free radicals can destroy healthy cells and tissues, and are believed to be a causal factor in many different diseases, ranging from Alzheimer's disease to cancer to heart disease. In fact, free radicals are a major culprit in the aging process itself! Our bodies produce antioxidants on their own, such as glutathione and Coenzyme Q 10. Vitamins C and E are well known antioxidant vitamins, but there are hundreds of other lesser-known but nevertheless important antioxidants found in herbs, as you will read in this book.

Thousands of years ago, when people first began using herbs, they had no idea why they worked. All they knew was that a certain plant elicited a desired result. When our ancestors first used foxglove to treat heart failure, they didn't know that this fuchsia-flowered plant contained molecules called *glycosides* that stimulate heart cells. When mothers in the Middle Ages soothed a scraped knee with a comfrey leaf, they didn't know that the plant's astringent tannins formed a protective surface over the wound, thus promoting healing. When Chinese healers prescribed licorice for arthritis flare-ups, they didn't know that it contained *saponins,* anti-inflammatory compounds similar to natural steroid hormones. When the Ancient Egyptians fed garlic to their slaves

CAUTION!

Just because herbs are natural substances doesn't mean that they can be used indiscriminately. Herbs can be strong medicine. Before trying any herbal remedy, be sure that you know what it does, how to use it, and the possible side effects. Never exceed the recommended dose. As a general rule, few medical problems occur from ingesting herbal remedies, but the potential for an allergic or toxic reaction is always there. In addition, about 1 percent of all plants are poisonous—mushrooms are a good example. Therefore, I do not recommend that people gather their own herbs unless they are skilled botanists. That's not to say that you cannot use the fresh dill, chives, or aloe from your garden or window box. Just don't consume anything that you are unsure of. Pregnant women should take herbs only under the direction of a knowledgeable physician or midwife. Not all herbs are safe for children; throughout the *Herb Bible* I advise parents as to which herbs can be used for children, and which should be avoided. Ideally, parents should check with a qualified health-care practitioner before giving any herb or over the counter medication to children.

to keep them healthy, they didn't know that it contained volatile oils that fight infection.

Thanks to modern laboratory techniques, we now understand how many of these herbs function. We are able to break down each plant into its basic molecular structure and analyze its extracts. Although we know a great deal more than our ancestors did about how some herbs work, there are still many more that need to be researched. Due to the lack of scientific data for many herbs, we must still rely heavily on information transmitted through folklore, antique herbals, and word of mouth. Ironically, we are only just discovering the scientific basis for many herbs that have been used successfully for millennia.

◾ How to Buy Herbs

In the past, if you wanted to use an herbal remedy, you had two choices: You could either grow your own or try to find it in the wild. And that was just the beginning of your labor. Once you found it, you had to pick it, dry it, grind it, boil it, or mix it in an alcohol solution to create a potent remedy. Needless to say, the process was extremely time consuming. In addition, due to differences in climate and growing conditions, you could never be absolutely sure that the plant you picked contained enough of the right active ingredients or that you had processed it in just the right way.

Today, you don't have to be a gardener or a chemist to use herbs safely and effectively. Herbs are now packaged in easy-to-use forms that eliminate much of the work and the guesswork. Several companies that have been making and selling vitamins for years now have their own lines of herb products and offer a standardized, guaranteed-potency product. This means that herbs sold by these and other reputable companies contain uniform levels of the compound or compounds believed to be responsible for the plant's medicinal activity, and that the herb is grown under safe conditions. Typically, these products are certified by an outside laboratory. There have been numerous reports in the press of packaged herbal products containing little, if any, of the herb or its active ingredients. These products will not work and are a waste of money. Therefore, it is extremely important that you buy standardized herbal extracts from reputable companies.

Look for products that have safety seals and are packaged in tamperproof bottles or boxes.

Because of the concern over pesticides and processing techniques, many manufacturers offer organically grown, nonirradiated products. There are times in the *Herb Bible* when I will recommend fresh herbs, but only in cases where they are easily accessible. In most cases, however, I recommend using a commercial herbal preparation.

Is it better to buy herbs in an herb shop than in a health food store? It all depends on what you're looking for. As a rule, herb shops carry a greater selection of dried herbs and teas, including many of the more exotic varieties. Although visiting an herb shop is a wonderful way to spend an afternoon, a well-stocked health food store may actually offer a better selection of prepared herbal remedies. It is also very difficult for the average consumer to assess the quality of goods in an herbal shop. If you don't live near an herb store or a health food store, or don't have time to shop, it is possible to buy herbs through the mail or the Internet.

Here is a list of some of the different ways
in which herbs are packaged and sold:

....

CAPSULES AND TABLETS.   Most of the commonly used herbs are now sold in capsule and tablet form, accounting for about two-thirds of all herb sales. The usual dose, depending on the herb, is 2 to 3 tablets or capsules, taken 2 to 3 times daily. Always follow the directions on the label.

EXTRACTS OR TINCTURES.   Extracts or tinctures are liquid herbal products, typically prepared by soaking herbs in an alcohol solution. However, there are some new alcohol-free extracts on the market that may be preferable in certain instances, especially for diabetics, pregnant women, children, and other people who should avoid alcohol. The usual dose, depending on the herb, is 10 to 30 drops, 2 to 3 times daily. Use as directed. Homeopathic extracts used by homeopathic practitioners are much stronger than conventional herbal tinctures and are strictly regulated by the FDA. They should be used only in conjunction with treatment by a homeopathic practitioner.

POWDERS. Some herbs are sold in powdered form. The required dose may be mixed in water or juice. If the herb is bitter, a drop of honey may be used as a sweetener. Some people, however, may prefer the convenience of capsules. Most stores will sell empty capsules, usually in number 0 size, that hold 400 to 450 mg. of herb. Kosher, gelatin-free capsules are available for vegetarians and people on restricted, religious diets.

DRIED HERBS. Dried herbs are sold in bulk, usually in large glass bottles. They should be stored in an airtight container at home, out of direct sunlight. These herbs may be put into capsules, but are usually brewed into a tea. It's very easy to do: Simply put 1 heaping tablespoon of herb into a tea ball or other infuser, and submerge it in 1 cup of hot water. Steep for 10 to 15 minutes. Drink the tea while it's hot. If you double the recipe, the leftover tea can be stored in the refrigerator and reheated. If you don't use a tea ball, you can put the dried herb directly into the hot liquid. When the tea is brewed, strain the liquid before drinking it.

PREPARED TEAS. Many herbs these days are sold in tea-bag form. Keep in mind that many of the teas you find in health food stores, especially those designated as "home remedies" for colds, are more potent than herbal tea sold in supermarkets and should only be used as directed.

NUTRACEUTICALS. *Nutraceuticals* are foods that have been fortified with herbs, vitamins, minerals, or other nutrients. Some herbs are sold in juice, nutrition bars, cereals, and even chips. They should be used according to package directions. The problem is, however, that the herbal ingredients may be so diluted, that they aren't effective. I would not use these products unless they specify the precise dose of the herb, and the active ingredients on their labels.

COMBINATION HERBAL PRODUCTS. A wide range of herbal remedies combining two or more herbs that work well together are available in capsule, tea, and extract form. For example, several herbs that are good for maintaining heart health, or herbs good for immune function, may be combined in one easy-to-use product. Use as directed.

CREAMS AND OINTMENTS. Many herbs that are commonly used externally are now sold commercially as creams and ointments. These preparations may have potent ingredients and should be used only as directed.

ESSENTIAL OILS. These are primarily used for bath oils, perfumes, massage oils, and for *aromatherapy,* the practice of using certain fragrances to promote health and relaxation. Essential oils are for external use only.

PERSONAL CARE. Several personal care product lines sell natural, pure, herbal products without any synthetic ingredients. These include herbal shampoos (not the herbal-scented shampoos you find in the supermarket), facial cleansers, deodorants, moisturizers, toothpaste, and even herbal mouthwash. There are also herbal cosmetic lines. These are excellent alternatives to chemical-laden products that can be potentially irritating for many people. An added plus is that many of these product lines are cruelty-free; that is, they are not tested on animals.

Shelf Life of Herbs

Dried herbs should be as fresh as possible. Try to buy them in a store with frequent turnover. Some packaged herbal products will have an expiration date printed on the package that will tell you when the herb is too stale to be useful. Unopened containers of tablets and capsules are usually good for up to two years. Keep your herbs in a cool, dark place out of direct heat or light. Once they are opened, dispose of them after one year.

Be an Alert Consumer

Unfortunately, there have been several disturbing stories in the natural food industry press about unscrupulous manufacturers or retailers who use a minute quantity of a particular herb and then market the product as a true herbal remedy or mislabel the product altogether. To ensure the quality of the product you are buying, purchase herbs sold by reputable companies. Look for the words "standardized herbal extract" on the label. If you have questions about a particular product line, call the manufacturer. Reliable companies welcome consumer inquiries. Get to know the owner of your local health food store or herb shop, and don't be afraid to ask questions. If you're buying herbs in bulk, find out who is supplying the store. If you don't understand the ingredients in a particular product, ask the owner to explain; most will be more than willing to share their knowledge and information with you.

New Labels

Recently, the Food and Drug Administration issued new labeling requirements for dietary supplements. Similar to the Nutrition Facts panel on food labels, nutritional supplements—all herbs, vitamins, minerals, and amino acids—must now have a Supplement Facts label. These new labels will detail the quantity of the main supplement or supplements included in the product, as well as a complete list of other ingredients. In the case of herbs, manufacturers will have to specify what part of the plant (root, leaf, or stem) has been used in the product.

Under the 1994 Dietary Supplement Health and Education Act, manufacturers of non-FDA–approved products like herbs are not allowed to make specific health claims. Therefore, manufacturers can only make vague references as to how to use these products. For example, manufacturers cannot say that a supplement is an effective treatment against arthritis; however, they can say that it promotes joint health. Clearly, it is more important than ever for supplement users to become educated consumers!

You may not see the new labels for some time. Manufacturers are allowed to sell out their existing stocks before being required to use the new labels.

Take the Right Amount

The amount of herb required for desired results may vary from person to person, depending on a number of factors. For example, a heavy person may require a larger dose than a very thin person. An older adult usually requires a smaller dose than a younger one. Regardless of age or weight, a person who is highly responsive to medications may require only a small amount of herb. To accommodate these differences, the recommended daily dose usually allows for some flexibility. For example, if, in the Hot Hundred, I advise you to mix between 10 and 30 drops of herbal extract in a cup of liquid, start with the lowest dose first to test for any adverse reaction. If the herb agrees with you, you may gradually work your way up to the maximum dose, if need be. However, if you are taking an herb for a particular problem, such as arthritics pain, and you find relief with the lower dose, there's no reason to increase it. Be very careful not to exceed the recommended dosages stated on the labels. Also, be aware that some herbs should be taken only for brief periods of time for a particular problem and are not safe for long-term use. Make sure that you learn as much as possible about any herb before taking it.

The Best Time to Take Herbal Remedies

Some people may feel nauseated if they take herbs on an empty stomach. If you use herbs on a daily basis, wait until after meals to take them. If you're using an herb for a specific problem, such as menstrual cramps or headache, take the herb as needed.

Use your common sense: Don't take a stimulating herb at night when you want to wind down. Don't take an herb that makes you sleepy before going to work or driving.

A Brief History of Herbal Medicine

The practice of herbal medicine may predate the human race. Animal behaviorists have observed that many animals instinctively seek specific plants when they are sick. As anyone who has ever cared for a dog knows, when the dog eats grass, it means that he probably has a stomachache. Early humans may have learned about the healing power of plants by mimicking this kind of animal behavior.

The first herbal guide dates back five thousand years, to the Sumerians, who used herbs such as caraway and thyme for healing. *Ayurveda,* the traditional medicine of India, still practiced today, may be even older. Herbal prescriptions were written in hieroglyphics on papyrus in ancient Egypt. Onions and garlic were favorite remedies. The first Chinese herbal, the *Wu Shi Er Bing Fang (Prescriptions for Fifty-two Diseases),* was compiled somewhere between 1065 and 711 B.C.E. It included herbs such as licorice, ginger, and astragalus root, which are all listed in the Hot Hundred! The Bible is full of references to herbs such as aloe, myrrh, and frankincense.

The Greek physician Hippocrates, who is believed to be the first practicing physician, recorded between three hundred and four hundred plant remedies in his writings. In the first century, another Greek physician, Dioscorides, listed five hundred plant medicines in his herbal, *De Materia Medica,* which was used until the seventeenth century. Galen, a famous physician who ministered to a Roman emperor and his gladiators, used a blend of herbs and magic to cure patients.

During the Middle Ages, ancient herbal remedies were passed on from generation to generation, but there was no uniform system of healing. A woman with a gynecological problem might seek help from the village wise woman, who had learned the art of herbal healing from another woman. The more affluent might seek care from a doctor who would prescribe his own homemade concoction made from plant or animal parts. Although the Catholic Church emphasized faith healing over other forms of healing, local monks preserved many of the early Greek and Roman medical texts. Many monasteries grew their own herbs and used them to treat their parishioners.

In the fifteenth century, the development of the printing press made information more accessible to the masses. John Gerard, a physician to the Tudor family, published *The Herball or General Historie of Plantes* in 1597; it was one of the first English herbals. It was quickly followed by Nicholas Culpeper's *The English Physician Enlarged,* an interesting blend of folklore, astrology, and botanical medicine. Both books became extremely popular and are still quoted by herbalists today.

When English settlers arrived in the New World, they exported their knowledge of herbal medicine, which they shared with the Native Americans. Native Americans, in turn, introduced the settlers to many local herbs that were then brought back to Europe, such as echinacea and goldenseal.

By the 1800s, the Western medical establishment began to turn to chemotherapy, the use of chemical drugs such as mercury, arsenic, and sulphur to cure disease. Herbal medicine, however, continued to be practiced by people who either couldn't afford conventional medical care or who preferred it over modern medical practices. In the United States, the Eclectics, a group of physicians who were prominent until the 1930s, still favored plant medicines, but they were a dying breed. Only homeopathic physicians, who follow the teachings of eighteenth-century physician Samuel Hahnemann, and a handful of other holistic practitioners continue to rely primarily on drugs derived from plants or animals.

Today, herbal medicine is still the primary source of healthcare for 80 percent of the world's population. As Westerners become more global in outlook, there is renewed interest in the traditional healing practices of other nations.

Hippocrates: The Father of Modern Medicine

Historians know surprisingly little about the man who is revered as the father of medicine. In fact, we're not even certain of the exact dates of his birth and death. All we know is that Hippocrates was born sometime in the fourth century on the Greek island of Kos. He died around 377. During his lifetime, he was a well-respected physician and teacher. Hippocrates rejected the idea that evil spirits were responsible for disease, the prevailing notion of the day. Rather, he proposed the radical theory that illness was a result of the improper balance of bodily fluids that he called the *four humors,* blood, phlegm, yellow bile, and black bile. According to Hippocrates, the real culprit was a poor diet, which left residues in the body. The father of medicine advocated the use of diet and plant medicines to prevent and cure disease. The Hippocratic oath, which doctors still take today, was probably composed by a follower of Hippocrates in the fourth century.

The First "Wonder Drug"

The *Ebers Papyrus,* named after Egyptologist Georg Ebers, is a papyrus written around 1600 B.C.E. that refers to more than seven hundred plant medicines including peppermint, myrrh, and castor oil. This early medical text recommends applying a moldy piece of bread to open wounds. In 1928, thousands of years later, Sir Alexander Fleming noticed in his laboratory by pure happenstance that bread mold was a potent antibiotic. His observation led to the development of penicillin and spawned the era of "wonder drugs."

Nicholas Culpeper: A Man for All Seasons

Nicholas Culpeper earned the wrath of the English medical establishment after the publication of his two works, *The English Physician People's Herbal* and an English translation of the Latin *Pharmacopeia,* which, up until then, was not widely available to the public. A medical school drop-out, Culpeper opened an apothecary in 1640, where he dispensed his low-cost botanical medicines. Culpeper's iconoclastic approach to medicine and his willingness to share information with the people made him very popular with the public, but he was despised by the medical establishment. Critics were quick to dismiss Culpeper as a quack, because he incorporated astrology with healing. Despite the astrological references, Culpeper's knowledge of plant medicines and their uses showed a great deal of sophistication for his time. In 1927, Mrs. C. F. Leyel, founder of the Society of Herbalists in London, opened a shop called *Culpeper's* in memory of the great herbalist. To this day, Culpeper's is probably the best known herbal shop in the world.

The Hot Hundred

Almond
Aloe vera
Apple
Arnica
Artichoke
Ashwagandha
Asparagus
Astragalus
Basil
Bee propolis
Bilberry
Bitter melon
Black cohosh
Boswellia
Bromelain
Burdock
Butcher's broom
Capsicum
Carrot
Cat's claw
Celery
Chamomile
Club moss tea
Comfrey
Cordyceps
Cranberry
Dandelion
Devil's claw

Dong quai
Echinacea
Elderberry
Ephedra
Evening primrose
Eyebright
Fennel
Fenugreek
Feverfew
Fo-ti
Garcinia cambogia
Garlic
Ginger
Ginkgo
Asian ginseng
American ginseng
Siberian ginseng
Goldenseal
Gotu kola
Grapeseed extract
Green tea
Guarana
Guggulipid
Hawthorne
Horse chestnut
Kava kava
Kudzu
Lavender

Licorice
Maitake mushroom
Marigold
Marshmallow
Milk thistle
Muira puama
Neem
Stinging nettle
Oat Fiber
Olive leaf extract
Onion
Oregano
Osha
Papaya
Parsley
Passionflower
Pau d'arco
Peppermint
Pine-bark extract
Psyllium
Pygeum
Raspberry leaves

Red clover
Red yeast rice
Reishi mushroom
Rosemary
St. John's wort
Sarsaparilla
Saw palmetto
Shiitake mushroom
Skullcap
Slippery elm bark
Soybean
Spirulina
Suma
Tea-tree oil
Turmeric
Uva ursi
Valerian
Vitex
White willow bark
Yerba santa
Yohimbe
Yucca

CHAPTER 2

The Hot Hundred

Literally *thousands of* herbs are used throughout the world, far too many to list in a single book. In this chapter, I have narrowed the number down to the Hot Hundred, the herbs that I feel have the potential to make the most significant contributions to our lives. Many of these herbs offer treatments and remedies for the ailments that most concern us today. You may already be familiar with a number of these herbs, and some may even be in your kitchen cabinet. Others may seem a bit strange at first, but, as you learn more about them, they will seem no more exotic than the rows and rows of synthetic chemical remedies found in any modern pharmacy. All of these herbs can be found in herb shops or health food stores in easy-to-use forms. After reading this chapter, you will see how simple it can be to incorporate herbs into your life.

■ How to Use the Hot Hundred

For each of the herbs listed in the Hot Hundred, I have included specific instructions as to appropriate use. However, the capsule or tablet size, or strength of a particular herbal product, may vary from manufacturer to manufacturer. Therefore, if you buy a packaged herb that recommends a different dose, follow the directions on the label. Unless otherwise specified, herbal extracts and powders can be mixed in juice, water, or made into tea. (For information on how to make herbal tea, see page 162). They can be sweetened with honey to taste. Warm beverages are the drink of choice for colds, coughs, menstrual cramps, and at bedtime.

Under "Personal Advice" I have listed any experience I may have had with a particular herb myself, or other pertinent anecdotal material.

CAUTION

Some of the Hot Hundred herbs are reputed to have anticancer properties, and may even be used to treat some forms of cancer in the United States and abroad. Anyone who is receiving treatment for cancer should not discontinue conventional treatment or use any herbs in conjunction with their treatment unless they are under the direction of a qualified physician. Parents should not give herbs to children without first checking with a pediatrician. Pregnant women should not take any herbs without asking an obstetrician.

ALMOND

• *Prunus amygdalus* •

FACTS

If you find commercial soap products too drying, check your local health food store for facial soaps and cleansers derived from almond. The kernel from the almond plant provides us with one of the best cleansers Mother Nature has to offer. It is also an excellent emollient. A recent study suggests that almond oil may also help prevent heart disease. At the Health Research and Studies Center in Los Altos, California, almond oil was shown to lower serum cholesterol levels in people who consumed it in place of saturated fat. According to this study, almond oil was a more potent cholesterol-reducing agent than olive oil! More studies are needed to determine if almond oil should be part of a heart-healthy lifestyle.

POSSIBLE BENEFITS

- Cleansers made from almond help to remove excess oil and dirt from skin.
- Almond butter and oil can moisturize and soften skin.
- Almond oil shows promise as a potent cholesterol reducer.

HOW TO USE IT

A handful of almond meal makes a good face scrub.

Rub a few drops of almond oil directly into rough areas, such as hands and heels of feet.

ALOE VERA

• *Aloe barbadenis* •

I have perfumed my bed with myrrh, aloes and cinnamon.

—PROVERBS 7:17

FACTS

For more than 3,500 years, healers and physicians have touted the benefits of this fragrant desert lily. There are about two hundred species of this amazing plant, but the aloe vera, "true aloe" in Latin, is considered the most effective healer. The leaf of aloe contains the special gel or emollient that is often used in cosmetics and skin creams. Aloe gel is regarded as one of nature's best natural moisturizers. The bitter juice, which is extracted from the whole leaf, may be taken internally for digestive disorders. Two thousand years ago, the Greek physician Dioscorides wrote that aloe vera was an effective treatment for everything from constipation to burns to kidney ailments. Queen Cleopatra regarded the gel as a fountain of youth, and used it to preserve her skin against the ravages of the Egyptian sun. The Egyptians were also believed to have used the aloe plant in their embalming process. The Bible is full of references to aloe, and it is still widely used in Africa to heal burns and wounds. A recent study in the *Journal of Dermatological Surgery and Oncology* shows that aloe vera significantly speeded the healing process of patients who underwent facial dermabrasion (the removal of the top layers of skin to remove scars). It is excellent for sunburns and other mild burns. Although most people have no adverse reactions to aloe vera skin products, people with highly sensitive skin may find aloe irritating. Always test an aloe product on a small patch of skin for 24 hours before using it on a larger surface.

A recent double-blind, placebo-controlled study performed in Sweden found that aloe vera cream (.5 percent strength) significantly improved symptoms in 83 percent of psoriasis patients when used three times a day for sixteen weeks. This is good news—psoriasis is not only difficult to treat, but since many of the conventional treatments for psoriasis are steroid based, they can only be used for a short time. If you have psoriasis, talk to your dermatologist to see whether aloe is a good choice for you.

Taken internally, aloe is a strong laxative. Frankly, I think there are kinder and gentler natural laxatives, such as psyllium, so I don't recommend aloe for this purpose.

Recently, *acemannan,* a compound extracted from aloe, has been shown to increase disease-fighting immune cells in mice whose immune systems had been compromised by exposure to radiation. Other studies suggest that acemannan may enhance the effect of AZT and acyclovir in blocking the spread of the AIDS virus. Obviously, a substance that both boosts immunity and helps prevent the spread of HIV would be an ideal treatment for AIDS patients along with other therapies. Time will tell whether this ancient herb can be an effective treatment for this modern-day ailment.

Researchers at Baylor College of Dentistry in Texas have reported that a gel made from acemannan helped promote the healing of oral ulcers better than conventional treatments.

POSSIBLE BENEFITS

- Soothes and promotes healing of sunburn and other minor burns.
- Useful for bug bites and mild skin irritations.

- Helps keep skin soft and supple.
- Acemannan, a compound from aloe gel, is an immune booster.

HOW TO USE IT

Aloe vera gel may be used liberally as needed.
Squeeze the fresh leaf and apply the liquid directly to affected area.

CAUTION: Do not take aloe internally during pregnancy. Aloe should not be used internally by children or the elderly.

Personal Advice

There are many so-called aloe vera preparations on the market that contain very little of this precious herb. Some contain only a minute quantity of aloe; others contain aloe extract, or reconstituted aloe vera, watered down versions that are not as beneficial as bonafide aloe gel. A true aloe product should list aloe vera as a primary ingredient (the first or second ingredient listed on the label) or state that it is 97 to 99 percent pure aloe vera.

APPLE

• *Pyrus malus* •

FACTS

The adage "An apple a day keeps the doctor away" may very well be true. In the second century, Galen, the famous court physician to emperors and gladiators, prescribed apple wine as a cure-all for nearly every ailment. While I wouldn't go quite that far in endorsing this fruit, I believe that apples can be an important part of your daily diet.

Apples are rich in *flavonoids,* disease-fighting compounds found in plants. Since 1965, researchers at Finland's Public Health Institute followed the dietary habits of 9,959 then cancer-free men and women between the ages of fifteen and ninety-nine. By 1991, 997 cases of cancer had been diagnosed, 151 of which were lung cancer. On close examination of the dietary differences between those who developed cancer and those who remained cancer-free, there was one striking difference. People who routinely ate foods rich in flavonoids were 20 percent less likely to develop cancer than those who did not. In fact, flavonoid eaters were at a 46 percent reduced risk of developing lung cancer. Of all the flavonoid-rich foods included in the diet, apples were found to be highly protective against cancer.

Quercetin is a type of flavonoid found in apples that may protect against cataracts. In animal studies, quercetin protected animals against cataracts even when they were exposed to chemicals that induce cataract formation.

Apples are also good for digestion. Depending on how they are used, they can relieve both constipation and diarrhea. Apples are also rich in *soluble fiber,* a substance that helps regulate blood sugar, preventing a sudden increase or drop in serum-sugar levels. *Pectin,* a type of soluble fiber found in apples, has received much attention lately because of its ability to lower blood cholesterol levels, thus reducing the risk of heart disease. Apples also are a traditional remedy for rheumatoid arthritis.

POSSIBLE BENEFITS
- May protect against cancer in general and lung cancer in particular.
- Helps regulate normal bowel function.
- Helps prevent both diarrhea and constipation.
- Reduces cholesterol and normalizes blood sugar.
- Traditional remedy for joint pain and stiffness due to rheumatism.

HOW TO USE IT
For diarrhea, eat a grated, peeled apple. Dried apple peels simmered in warm water help regulate digestion. For maximum benefit, eat 1 to 2 medium apples every day.

ARNICA
....
• *Arnica montana* •

F A C T S

The flower and root of this plant have been used by natural healers as a pain reliever, expectorant, and stimulant. Modern herbalists, however, believe that arnica is very strong medicine, and should not be taken internally unless it is in the much weakened homeopathic form (Dose 10–30X) under the supervision of a homeopathic physician. An overdose can be fatal. Rubbed on the skin, however, arnica is wonderful for healing bruises or other skin irritations. Use only on unbroken skin. Commercially prepared liniments may also be used for muscle soreness or arthritis.

POSSIBLE BENEFITS
- Soothes and heals skin wounds and irritations.
- Relieves pain due to muscle spasm or joint inflammation.
- Used internally, it's good for coughs, but use only under the supervision of a homeopathic physician.

HOW TO USE IT
There are several commercially prepared salves or ointments that are safe to use externally as needed. An ointment that is too strong will cause further irritation. Therefore, I do not recommend that people prepare their own salves.

CAUTION: Never apply arnica to broken skin. If further irritation develops, discontinue use. Never take arnica internally unless it is under the supervision of a physician.

ARTICHOKE
• *Cynara scolymus* •

FACTS

The flower or head of the artichoke, commonly known as the *heart,* is reputed to be an aphrodisiac, although this claim has never been scientifically proven. Even if this popular vegetable is not good for affairs of the heart, it is certainly good for the heart itself. Through the years, various studies worldwide have shown that people's blood cholesterol levels dropped after eating artichoke. In fact, an anticholesterol drug called *cynara* is derived from this herb. In 1940, a study in Japan showed that artichoke not only reduced cholesterol but it also increased bile production by the liver and worked as a good diuretic.

Artichoke concentrate is now available in capsules at natural food stores. In a recent multicenter study involving more than 550 patients, those taking an average of 1.5 grams of artichoke leaf extract daily showed a major decline in both total cholesterol and triglycerides within six weeks. Other studies have shown that artichoke extract boosts levels of HDL or "good" cholesterol. Researchers suspect that artichoke works by both reducing cholesterol production by the liver and helping the body better eliminate excess cholesterol.

Similar to its relative, milk thistle, artichoke also appears to have a protective effect on the liver.

POSSIBLE BENEFITS
- Relieves excess water weight.
- Promotes heart health by reducing cholesterol.
- Enhances liver function.

HOW TO USE IT
Take four 500 mg. capsules daily.

To make a delicious, heart-healthy treat, rub an artichoke with olive oil and tuck a few slices of garlic in the leaves. Steam for 30 to 40 minutes. Remember that the benefits of this vegetable will be lost if you douse it in melted butter, which is high in saturated fat, or in margarine, which is high in calories.

ASHWAGANDHA

• *Withania somnifera* •

FACTS

In Sanskrit, *ashwagandha* means "that which has the smell of a horse." The root of this herb does indeed smell like a horse, but that hasn't stopped it from becoming one of the most sought-after herbs in India for more than 1000 years, or from gaining a newfound popularity in the United States. Known as *Indian ginseng,* ashwagandha is used as a tonic, primarily for men. It is reputed to restore energy, vitality, and mental function. Ashwagandha is a well-known aphrodisiac, touted for its ability to enhance sex drive and improve erectile function. Animal studies show that, similar to ginseng, ashwagandha can increase stamina and bolster physical performance in mice, which suggests that it may have a similar effect in humans. Laboratory studies show that ashwagandha contains potent immune boosters that bolster the body's ability to weed out cancerous cells.

Ayurvedic physicians prescribe ashwagandha to men and women who suffer from chronic or debilitating illness. A natural anti-inflammatory, ashwagandha is also used to treat arthritis, usually in combination with other anti-inflammatories, such as boswellia (see page 50).

POSSIBLE BENEFITS
- Increases strength and vitality.
- Helps the body to fight disease.
- Sexual rejuvenator for men.
- Relieves symptoms of arthritis.

HOW TO USE IT

Take up to three 4.5 mg. standardized tablets daily.

ASPARAGUS
• *Asparagus officinalis* •

FACTS

Asparagus is a highly regarded herb worldwide. Chinese pharmacists save the best roots of the asparagus plant for their families and friends in the belief that it will increase feelings of compassion and love. In India, this herb is used to promote fertility, reduce menstrual cramping, and increase milk production in nursing mothers. In the Western world, it has been touted as an aphrodisiac. These customs and beliefs are not mere superstition: Asparagus root contains compounds called *steroidal glycosides* that directly affect hormone production, and may very well influence emotions. An excellent diuretic, asparagus is also very nutritious. It is high in folic acid, which is essential for the production of new red-blood cells. Many herbal healers recommend asparagus root for rheumatism, due to the anti-inflammatory action of steroidal glycosides. Powdered seed from the asparagus plant is good for calming an upset stomach.

POSSIBLE BENEFITS
- Stimulates hormone production.
- Helps rid the body of excess water and salt.
- Helps prevent anemia due to folic acid deficiency.
- Soothes pain and swelling of joints due to rheumatism or arthritis.

HOW TO USE IT

Eat the young shoots and seeds. The seed is available in powder form. Take 1 teaspoon powder daily in juice.

CAUTION: Do not use if your kidneys are inflamed; asparagus increases the rate of urinary production.

ASTRAGALUS

• *Astragalus membranaceous* •

FACTS

Asian herbalists have used astragalus, grown in China for centuries, for a wide variety of ailments, including diabetes, heart disease, and high blood pressure. Westerners, however, are just beginning to discover its many benefits. Recent studies in leading Chinese medical journals suggest that astragalus may help activate the immune system, thus enhancing the body's natural ability to fight disease. Astragalus may also prevent the spread of malignant cancer cells to healthy tissue. Researchers at the University of Texas in Houston found that an extract from this plant helped restore normal immune function in cancer patients with impaired immunity. Although chemotherapy and radiation kill cancer cells, in the process, these treatments can leave the body weakened and more susceptible to infection. Some herbalists routinely give astragalus to people undergoing chemotherapy and radiation. In particular, astragalus boosts the production and effectiveness of immune cells, which fight viruses and tumors. More research is underway to explore the full medical potential of this ancient cure-all. Modern herbalists recommend taking astragalus to help ward off colds and flus.

POSSIBLE BENEFITS
- Promotes resistance to disease.
- Mild stimulant.
- May reduce blood pressure by helping to rid the body of excess water weight.

- May help improve immune function for cancer patients.

HOW TO USE IT

Take up to three 400 mg capsules daily.

CAUTION: If you are undergoing chemotherapy, do not take astragalus (or any other medication) without first consulting a doctor who is familiar with this herb.

The Heart Herb

In 1775, English physician William Withering diagnosed a patient with congestive heart failure as hopeless and sent him home to die. A short time later, he learned that a local folk healer had cured the patient using a bunch of mysterious herbs. Amazed by the man's miraculous recovery, Withering investigated the herbs used by the healer and isolated foxglove Digitalis purpurea as the main ingredient. After performing several experiments, Withering discovered that this purple-flowered plant was a potent cardiotonic, that is, it improved the heart's pumping action, helping to rid the body of the excess fluid causing the congestion. Withering also learned that in the wrong dose, foxglove could be lethal, triggering a fatal arrhythmia or irregularity in the heartbeat. For the next decade, Withering conducted numerous experiments to determine the precise amount of this drug needed to treat heart failure. He published his results in 1785, informing other physicians of this amazing new cure. Today, *digitalis,* the drug derived from foxglove, is a highly regarded treatment for heart failure. Due to its unpredictable effect on the heart, the herb should never be consumed without a doctor's supervision.

BASIL

• *Ocimum basilicum* •

FACTS

The word *basil* is derived from the Greek word for *king*, suggesting that the ancient healers held this aromatic plant in high regard. Today we think of basil as something that you either sprinkle over tomato sauce or pound into a pesto. Fresh basil is delicious to eat, but the herb is also an effective remedy for a variety of digestive disorders, including stomach cramps, vomiting, and constipation.

POSSIBLE BENEFITS

- Reduces stomach cramps and nausea.
- Relieves gas.
- Promotes normal bowel function.
- Aids digestion.

HOW TO USE IT

Mix 1 teaspoon of dried herbs in 1/2 cup of warm water. Strain. Drink 1 to 2 cups as needed daily.

BEE PROPOLIS

FACTS

Much of what we know about herbal medicine was learned by observing how animals protected themselves against the same microscopic predators that stalk humans—viruses, fungi, and bacteria. For centuries, herbalists have been fascinated by how bees fortify their hives against intruders and unwanted infections. Bees seal their hives with a sticky substance known as *propolis* or *bee glue*, which is collected from plants. Insects or small animals caught in the hive are first stung into submission, then immobilized by the propolis but, interestingly, their bodies do not decay. If they did, they would spread infection throughout the hive. Ancient healers such as Hippocrates deduced that bee propolis must have special disinfectant properties, and prescribed it for skin wounds and stomach ulcers. Propolis was used to treat wounds on the battlefield during World War I, the pre-antibiotic age, and during World War II, when penicillin was scarce.

Scientific studies confirm that once again, Hippocrates was way ahead of his time. Compounds in propolis have been shown to be effective against a wide range of disease producing microbes, including *staphylococcus aureus MRSA,* a leading cause of staph infection in hospitals. Since many forms of staph are now antibiotic resistant, propolis may be just what the doctor ordered to reduce the risk of infection during hospital stays. (About 10 percent of all hospital patients develop some form of infection while they are in the hospital.) Propolis is rich in bioflavonoids, vitamins, and minerals. In addition to fighting infection on the outside of the body, propolis can also boost the body's ability to fight disease on the inside. Used as a gargle, it can relieve a raw sore throat while promoting healing.

POSSIBLE BENEFITS

- Heals skin wounds, relieves pain from herpes lesions, and promotes healing.
- Propolis salve and mouthwash can fight gum infections and sore throats.
- Effective against disease-causing microorganisms.

HOW TO USE IT

For external use, use propolis skin creams and ointments as directed. For internal use, use propolis salve for sore and infected gums.

At the first sign of a cold, slowly dissolve a zinc lozenge that includes propolis, vitamin C, echinacea, and goldenseal in your mouth.

To boost immunity, take one 200 mg. tablet daily.

BILBERRY

• *Vaccinium myrtillus* •

FACTS

Bilberry, a European relative of the blueberry, is a well-known folk remedy for poor vision, especially for people who suffer from *night blindness*, that is, they have difficulty seeing in the dark. In fact, legend has it, bilberry jam was given to Royal Air Force pilots who flew nighttime missions during World War II. Bilberry contains *anthocyanidins*, phytochemicals that are potent antioxidants that protect the eyes from free-radical damage due to exposure to UV light from sun and pollution. Anthocyanidin may help improve the microcirculation to the eye by protecting small blood vessels from free-radical attack. Bilberry works by accelerating the regeneration of retinol purple, commonly known as *visual purple*, a substance required for good eyesight. European medical journals are filled with studies confirming bilberry's positive effect on vision.

POSSIBLE BENEFITS

- Helps preserve eyesight and prevent eye damage.
- Particularly useful for people who suffer from eyestrain or poor night vision.
- Good for people who must drive at night.
- Helpful for nearsightedness.

HOW TO USE IT

Take 1 60 mg. capsule up to 4 times daily.
Mix 15 to 40 drops of extract in water or juice, and drink 3 times daily.

BITTER MELON

• *Momordica chirantia* •

FACTS

The current bestselling book *Sugar Busters* warns that the sugar-laden American diet is leading us down the road to obesity and disease. It's no secret that a diet rich in overly processed, refined carbohydrates and junk food can lead to insulin resistance and Type II diabetes. Insulin is the hormone that breaks sugar down into a form that can be used by the body's cells. Unlike Type I diabetes, which is caused by a lack of insulin, in Type II diabetes, the body produces plenty of insulin, but the cells have grown resistant to it. Type II diabetes is a virtual epidemic in the United States. If untreated, diabetes can lead to serious problems, including heart disease, nerve damage, kidney damage, and blindness. The good news is that herbs such as bitter melon can help control the problem.

For centuries, Ayurvedic physicians have used bitter melon, often along with other herbs, to treat Type II diabetes. Several studies show it can normalize blood-sugar levels in Type II diabetics, which has led researchers to suspect that it may work by either stimulating the release of insulin, or have an insulinlike effect on its own. Anyone who has diabetes should be treated by a knowledgeable physician or natural healer. A combination of the right diet, supplements, and exercise can control, and even reverse, diabetes in many cases.

It's interesting to note that, in Ayurvedic medicine, one herb often has numerous uses and bitter melon is no exception to this rule. Recently, bitter melon has been shown to stop the growth of HIV (the virus that causes AIDS) in test-tube studies. It appears to stimulate the production of disease-fighting immune cells. Many AIDS patients are already incorporating bitter melon into their treatment regimens under the supervision of nutritionally oriented physicians. Animal studies have shown bitter melon to be effective in controlling cancerous tumors, but whether it works as well in humans remains to be seen.

POSSIBLE BENEFITS
- Helps to control blood sugar.
- Enhances immune system.
- May be useful against HIV.

HOW TO USE IT
Take one 500 mg. capsule 30 minutes before each meal.

Personal Advice
For maximum benefit, drink eight glasses of water daily. Bitter melon should not be used by pregnant or lactating women.

BLACK COHOSH
• *Cimicifuga racemosa* •

FACTS

Native Americans used this herb to reduce the pain and inflammation of rheumatoid arthritis, and to treat an assortment of "women's disorders." Today, black cohosh is being touted as the herbal alternative to estrogen-replacement therapy, as well as a natural remedy for PMS and menstrual disorders. Studies performed in Europe have shown that black cohosh performs as well as estrogen in helping relieve both the physical and emotional symptoms associated with menopause, including hot flashes, insomnia, mild depression, and irritability. Black cohosh works by inhibiting the secretion of luteinizing hormone (LH), which is responsible for many of the unpleasant symptoms associated with menopause. In fact, black cohosh has received the stamp of approval from the German Commission E, the scientific board that evaluates the efficacy and safety of herbal treatments, for treatment of menopausal symptoms, PMS, and menstrual disorders. What isn't yet known is whether black cohosh can protect against heart disease and osteoporosis the way estrogen can. Nor do we know the long-term effects of using black cohosh. What we do know is that women have used this herb for several hundred years. In fact, at the turn of the century, one of the most popular female tonics was Lydia Pinkham's Vegetable Compound, which included a hefty dose of black cohosh!

Herbalists have also used black cohosh to treat persistent coughs in cases of asthma, bronchitis, and whooping cough.

POSSIBLE BENEFITS
- Relieves menopausal symptoms.
- Used as a muscle relaxant.
- Natural anti-inflammatory treatment for rheumatoid arthritis.

HOW TO USE IT
Take one 40 mg. capsule daily until symptoms are relieved; use for up to six months.
Mix 10 to 30 drops of extract in liquid daily.

CAUTION: Do not use during pregnancy until labor and only under the supervision of a doctor. Do not confuse with blue cohosh, which has not been as well studied and could be toxic in high doses.

BOSWELLIA
• *Boswellia serata* •

FACTS

The gummy resin of the boswellia serata plant has been used as a natural anti-inflammatory for thousands of years. Modern science has verified what ancient Ayurvedic healers knew all along: Boswellia is often an excellent treatment for arthritis. Several Indian studies report that, based on animal studies, compounds derived from boswellia, called *boswellic acids*, can reduce signs of inflammation in the knee joint. Boswellia blocks the formation of *leukotrienes*, immune cells that trigger inflammation and promote the formation of free radicals. It also improves the blood supply to joints, which helps keep the soft tissue nourished and viable. Another double-blind, placebo-controlled study conducted at the University of Poona in India found that osteoarthritis patients experienced significant reduction in symptoms after taking an herbal formula that contained ashwagandha, turmeric, and zinc complex. Patients reported a decrease in morning stiffness, as well as improved physical performance and grip strength.

Boswellia is not just good for sore joints; it can also protect against heart disease. Studies published in Indian medical journals report that boswellia extract can lower high cholesterol and high triglyceride levels, and have prevented or reversed the formation of clogged arteries in animals fed a high-fat diet.

Ayurvedic healers use boswellia for other conditions related to inflammation, including psoriasis, allergies, and ulcerative colitis.

POSSIBLE BENEFITS
- Soothes pain and swelling associated with arthritis.
- Controls inflammation and may help reduce symptoms of inflammatory diseases.

HOW TO USE IT
Boswellia creams and ointments can be rubbed direct on the affected joint, or boswellia can be taken orally in capsule form.
Take three 500 mg. capsules daily until symptoms subside, then reduce dose to one 500 mg. capsule daily.

BROMELAIN

FACTS

Nature's pharmacy is replete with substances that can help control *inflammation*, the process within the body that is a contributing if not the causal factor of numerous diseases, from arthritis to allergies to cancer.

Inflammation begins when the immune system detects a problem somewhere in the body and sends a legion of special cells, called *leukocytes,* to deal with it. Here's how the inflammatory process makes arthritis worse. Arthritis begins with the wearing down of cartilage, the substance that lines the joints, resulting in pain and swelling that interferes with the normal flow of blood. In response, the immune system produces leukocytes, which accumulate in the joint. The leukocytes attack what they perceive to be an enemy by producing *free radicals,* molecules that are highly reactive and can destroy disease cells as well as healthy tissue. The joint becomes inflamed, enlarged, and stiff. The best way to reduce these symptoms, short of regrowing the cartilage, is to control the inflammation. *Bromelain,* an enzyme derived from pineapple, can help. In fact, it is often included in special herbal formulas designed to control arthritis pain. Some studies suggest that bromelain is similar to *corticosteroids,* powerful drugs that inhibit inflammation, but have potentially dangerous side effects such as high blood pressure, elevated cholesterol, and wearing down of the bone. Unless the situation is life-threatening, it certainly makes sense to try herbal anti-inflammatories such as bromelain before resorting to corticosteroids.

People with arthritis often take nonsteroidal anti-inflammatories (such as ibuprofen or aspirin), which are effective in relieving pain, but can upset the stomach. Unlike commercial anti-inflammatories, bromelain is an excellent digestive aid. In fact, I often recommend bromelain tablets for people who have chronic indigestion.

Athletes use bromelain to help promote healing of sports injuries. It is also useful for treating bruises. Look for bromelain in herbal formulas for allergy symptoms, often combined with quercetin.

POSSIBLE BENEFITS
- Reduces inflammation associated with arthritis.
- Helps accelerate healing of injuries and wounds.
- May relieve allergic symptoms.

HOW TO USE IT

For arthritis or allergy, take one 500 mg. tablet or capsule twice daily at least two hours before or after eating. For indigestion, take one 500 mg. chewable tablet after meals.

BURDOCK

• *Arctium lappa* •

FACTS

Natural healers revere this herb as nature's best *blood purifier,* that is, they believe that it rids the body of dangerous toxins. Ancient herbalists used burdock to treat snake bites. Nicholas Culpeper, the famous seventeenth-century herbalist, wrote that it "helpeth those that are bit by a mad dog." Today, many herbalists still recommend this herb for its diuretic action: It increases the flow of urine and promotes sweating. It is also reputed to be helpful for the soreness and swelling caused by arthritis, rheumatism, sciatica, and lumbago. Used externally, it is considered a major natural treatment for skin problems such as eczema, psoriasis, and even canker sores. Burdock is also soothing for hemorrhoids.

POSSIBLE BENEFITS
- Helps rid body of excess water weight.
- Soothes pain caused by arthritis, rheumatism, and backache.
- Relieves skin irritation.

HOW TO USE IT

Take up to 3 capsules daily.
Mix 10 to 25 drops extract in liquid daily.
Apply locally to inflamed area as needed.

BUTCHER'S BROOM

• *Ruscus acluteatus* •

FACTS

In Europe, practitioners of folk medicine have relied on this herb for centuries to relieve excess water retention and constipation. Today, it is extremely popular among European women to treat the discomfort and pain caused by poor circulation in the legs—that heavy-leg feeling also known as *restless-leg syndrome*. French scientists discovered that this plant contains steroidal-type compounds that can constrict veins and reduce inflammation. Butcher's broom has also been used to soothe the swelling and pain of rheumatoid arthritis. Taken orally or made into an ointment, it is excellent for the treatment of hemorrhoids.

POSSIBLE BENEFITS
- Improves circulation in hands and feet.
- Helps reduce edema in legs or feet.
- Anti-inflammatory action can reduce swelling caused by arthritis and rheumatism.
- Reduces pain caused by hemorrhoids.

HOW TO USE IT
Take up to 3 capsules daily.
Mix 10 to 20 drops extract in liquid daily.
Apply small amounts of ointment to hemorrhoids until inflammation has cleared.

Personal Advice
This is a particularly good herb for people who are on their feet most of the day, such as salespersons, teachers, and doctors, who, as a result, experience swelling at night.

CAPSICUM OR CAYENNE

• *Capsicum frutescens* •

FACTS

Contrary to popular belief, hot, spicy food may actually be good for your health, that is, if it contains liberal amounts of cayenne, also known as *capsicum.* Cayenne is used as an overall digestive aid: It stimulates the production of gastric juices, improves metabolism, and even helps relieve gas. Cayenne is also very nutritious. Peppers in general contain more vitamin C than oranges, as well as iron, calcium, phosphorous, and B-complex vitamins. A meal rich in cayenne will have a mildly stimulating effect on the body.

Capsaicin is the substance in cayenne that gives the spice its kick. Capsaicin blocks the production of a chemical called *substance P,* which triggers pain and inflammation. Recently, capsaicin cream has been studied as a treatment for shingles or to reduce pain from diabetic neuropathy. Cayenne has been used successfully to treat patients with *cluster headaches,* a particularly painful type of headache.

Cayenne tea is excellent for a cold and chills. Cayenne also appears to have a beneficial effect on blood fats. According to a 1987 study published in the *Journal of Bioscience,* rats fed a diet high in cayenne experienced a significant reduction in blood triglycerides and low-density lipoproteins, or "bad" cholesterol. Thai researchers found a correlation between a diet rich in cayenne and a lower incidence of blood clots. Further studies have shown that cayenne helps break down blood clots efficiently.

POSSIBLE BENEFITS
- Helps relieve pain and inflammation.
- Digestive aid.
- Reduces discomfort caused by the common cold.
- Stimulates the appetite.

HOW TO USE IT

Take up to 3 capsules daily.

Drink one cup tea for stomach cramps or a cold daily.
Prepared teas are available, or make it from dried herb.

Rub cream or ointment on affected areas.

CAUTION: Cayenne can be irritating to hemorrhoids. It should not be used by people with gastrointestinal problems. Never apply cayenne ointment to broken skin. Prolonged application can cause skin irritation. If taking internally, do not exceed recommended dose. High dosages taken internally may cause gastroenteritis and kidney damage.

The Spice of Life

Some well-known herbs have spicy pasts. Caraway seeds were once used in love potions. Coriander, a popular ingredient in salsa, was once a highly regarded aphrodisiac. Even the common onion was at one time prescribed by herbalists to restore sexual potency.

CARROT

• *Daucus carota* •

FACTS

Was Bugs Bunny an early practitioner of preventive medicine? His favorite snack was carrots, a rich source of *carotenoids,* chemicals found in plants which are now being studied for their cancer-fighting activity. One carotenoid abundant in carrots, *alpha carotene,* has been shown to suppress the growth of cancerous tumors in animals. Another carotenoid found in carrots, *beta carotene,* may reduce the risk of both cancer and cardiovascular disease. Carrots are a member of the *umbelliferae* family (along with celery and parsnips), which are being investigated by the National Cancer Institute for potential health benefits. Numerous studies worldwide confirm that people who eat diets high in carrots and other foods rich in carotene are less likely to develop certain forms of cancer than those who don't. In fact, studies show that even people who are exposed to specific carcinogens, such as tobacco and ultraviolet light, could reduce their risk of cancer by eating more carotene.

Carrots contain *calcium pectate,* a type of soluble fiber shown to reduce blood-cholesterol levels. Two carrots a day may reduce cholesterol levels by as much 20 percent in people with high cholesterol!

The RDA recommended daily allowance for carotenoids is 5,000 IU, but cancer researchers suggest that in order to dramatically decrease your cancer risk, you should consume about 12,500 IU per day. This isn't too difficult, considering that one grated, raw carrot daily provides about 13,500 units of carotene.

Carotenoids are also excellent for the eyes. Beta carotene permits the formation of visual purple in the eyes, which helps counteract night blindness and weak vision. Carrots are also a good treatment for diarrhea, and can relieve gas and heartburn.

POSSIBLE BENEFITS
- Promotes eye health.
- Helps prevent cancer.
- Lowers cholesterol.
- Soothes indigestion.
- Can help relieve diarrhea.

HOW TO USE IT
Drink 1 to 2 cups homemade carrot juice daily, if you have an automatic juicer, or commercially prepared fresh product.

Personal Advice

When it comes to carrots, the fresher the product the better. From the minute the carrot is picked, the carotene begins to lose its potency. Try to buy loose carrots from the greengrocer and avoid the stuff that's sold in plastic bags. Use them as quickly as possible.

If you don't like carrots, there are new supplements on the market containing mixtures of carotenoids extracted from vegetables. Although they don't contain fiber like real carrots do, carotenoid capsules are an easy way for non-carrot eaters to get some carotenoids into their diet. In my opinion, fresh carrots are still your best bet!

CAT'S CLAW
• *Uncaria tornentosa* •

FACTS

Also known by its Spanish name, *uña de gato,* this herb grows wild in the Peruvian Amazon. Indians native to that region have used it for hundreds of years to treat immune disorders and digestive problems. Recently, cat's claw has become a superstar among herbs because of its reputation as an immune booster that can help slow down the progress of the AIDS virus. What is particularly insidious about the AIDS virus is that it knocks out the immune system's disease-fighting T cells, in effect crippling the body's ability to fight infection. According to a small study reported in 1993 in a Peruvian newspaper, five out of seven AIDS patients taking a cat's claw extract showed an increase in T cells, as well as overall improvement. However, cat's claw did not work for everyone, nor did the physician conducting the study claim it was a cure for AIDS. At best, it is a useful tool to be used along with other therapies. European researchers are using cat's claw in conjunction with AZT, a standard drug therapy for AIDS.

Cat's claw has also been touted as a potential cancer treatment. In 1988, Peruvian physicians at the International Congress on Traditional Medicines in Lima reported success in treating hundreds of cancer patients with cat's claw. Although innovative physicians have incorporated cat's claw in their treatment of cancer, there have not been any clinical trials to determine its effectiveness. Although it makes sense that an immune-enhancing agent would help the body fight against cancer (as well as other less serious diseases), for a life-threatening illness such as cancer, I recommend using herbs and other alternative treatments only in conjunction with conventional medicine. Until all the facts are in, you don't want to gamble with your life! On the other hand, if you're looking for an immune booster to help ward off colds and flu, cat's claw may be just what your immune system needs to get you through the winter.

Recently, scientists have isolated a natural anti-inflammatory in cat's claw that is reputed to be effective against arthritis. It is now included in many herbal arthritis formulas.

POSSIBLE BENEFITS
- Bolsters immune system.
- Anti-inflammatory.

HOW TO USE IT
Take up to three 500 mg. capsules daily.

CELERY

• *Apium graveolens* •

FACTS

Although you may think of celery as nothing more than something crunchy to chop into a salad, the root, leaves, and seeds of this plant offer many health benefits. Scientists at the University of Chicago have discovered that celery contains a chemical called *3-butylphthalide,* which reduces blood pressure in animals. Chinese healers have used celery for centuries as a treatment for high blood pressure. Celery juice and extract of celery seed are excellent diuretics that promote the flow of urine through the kidneys. Celery has a calming effect on the digestive system, relieving gas and indigestion. It is also reputed to be helpful against rheumatoid arthritis and gout.

POSSIBLE BENEFITS

- Natural diuretic.
- May lower blood pressure.
- Good for digestion system and enhances appetite.
- May relieve symptoms of rheumatism and gout.

HOW TO USE IT

Take 1 tablespoon juice 2 to 3 times daily.
Mix 6 to 8 drops celery oil in water, and drink twice
    daily.

CAUTION: Celery juice and oil should not be used during pregnancy.

CHAMOMILE OR CAMOMILE
• *Matricaria chamomilla* •

FACTS

Back in the days when women often came down with a mysterious malady called *the vapors,* a cup of chamomile tea was often prescribed to relieve female anxiety. Known for its calming effect on smooth muscle tissue, chamomile is still a popular remedy for nervous stomach, menstrual cramps, and other common problems often related to stress. Since 1600, Europeans have used chamomile as a cure for insomnia, neuralgia, back pain, and rheumatoid arthritis. They were not the first to discover this herb; ancient Egyptians included chamomile in their arsenal of herbal cures.

Chamomile contains natural anti-inflammatories including *apigenin,* which is similar in action to that of non asteroidal anti-inflammatories (NSAIDS.) Its natural antispasmodic compounds can calm an irritated stomach. Chamomile also contains chemicals that are antibacterial and antifungal. Chamomile is very soothing to the skin and is included in skin creams and cleansers. Used externally chamomile cream is also good for skin inflammations and sunburns. It is particularly good for people with sensitive skin. Used as a mouthwash, chamomile tea can relieve the pain of toothache. Chamomile extract is put in shampoos to enhance golden highlights of blond hair. A cup of chamomile tea is a perfect nightcap.

POSSIBLE BENEFITS

- Good for the digestion.
- Has a relaxing effect on the body.
- Traditional treatment for rheumatoid arthritis.
- Relieves back pain.
- Soothes skin irritations.
- Good for sunburn.

HOW TO USE IT

Take up to 3 capsules daily.
Mix 10 to 20 drops extract in water up to 3 times daily.
Drink 1 cup tea daily.
Rub extract on skin irritations as needed. Put a few
    drops of chamomile oil in bath water to relieve
    hemorrhoids.

CAUTION: Chamomile is a member of the daisy family, and anyone who is allergic to other members of the daisy family, including ragweed, should steer clear of this herb. If you are unsure, consult your doctor or allergist.

Personal Advice

I drink a cup nightly as a sleep aid. In restaurants, chamomile tea is often available instead of regular tea, which contains caffeine.

CLUB MOSS TEA
....
• *Hupersia serrata* •

FACTS

If you were an older person who lived in China today and were experiencing memory problems, you would visit your local herbal healer. He or she would then concoct a special tea that would undoubtedly include an Asian variety of club moss. Although club moss has been used in traditional Chinese medicine for several centuries—and still is—scientists have only recently discovered the scientific basis behind the folklore. Club moss contains two chemicals—*huperzine A* and *huperzine B*—which, in mice, have been shown to improve learning, memory retrieval, and memory retention. Based on anecdotal evidence and its long use in Chinese medicine, it would appear that these chemicals have similar effects on two-legged animals.

Huperzine inhibits the action of an enzyme that breaks down *acetylcholine,* a neurotransmitter that is essential for memory. People with dementia often have lower-than-normal levels of acetylcholine, which may hamper their ability to retain information.

POSSIBLE BENEFITS
• Memory booster.

HOW TO USE IT
Drink 1 cup of club moss tea daily. It is also available in tablet or capsule form in combination with other herbs such as ginkgo biloba, plus brain-boosting supplements such as DMAE, phosphatidyl choline, inositol, and serine. Take up to 3 tablets daily or follow directions on the label.

COMFREY

• *Symphytum officinale* •

FACTS

Generations of herbal healers have used comfrey to treat skin wounds without knowing why this plant is so effective. We now know that comfrey contains *allantoin,* a substance that helps stimulate the growth of new cells and is now used in many cosmetic products. Commercially prepared comfrey creams and ointments are useful for all kinds of skin irritations, including chafing and bug bites. External comfrey preparations have also been used to promote healing of damaged tendons or ligaments.

At one time, comfrey was taken internally for ulcers and irritable bowel syndrome. Today, we are more cautious about ingesting comfrey, because it contains *pyrroliziidine alkaloids,* compounds known to cause liver disease if taken over a long period of time. In 1978, the National Cancer Institute reported that rats fed comfrey roots or leaves developed liver cancer. In fact, in the 1980s, two medical journals— *Gastroenterology* in the United States, and the *British Medical Journal*— reported two cases of liver damage resulting from the frequent consumption of comfrey-pepsin tablets for gastrointestinal disorders. In Canada, Russian comfrey, which contains high levels of pyrroliziidine, has been banned. Common comfrey, which contains much lower levels of this dangerous substance, is still sold freely.

In the United States, the FDA is investigating pyrroliziidine alkaloid levels in domestic comfrey. Due to its potential cancer hazard, the internal use of comfrey is a controversial subject among herbalists. Some believe that it should never be ingested. Others, however, feel that in low doses it is harmless as compared to other substances. Proponents of comfrey cite a 1987 study reported in *Science* magazine that rated carcinogens based on their potential risk. Noted carcinogen authority Bruce Ames of the University of California estimated that one cup of comfrey tea was about as risky as eating one peanut butter sandwich, which has traces of *estragole,* a natural carcinogen. In light of the uncertainty over its safety, however, I believe that comfrey should not be taken internally, especially since there are other safer herbs that can be used in its place, such as peppermint, balm, and ginger.

POSSIBLE BENEFITS
- Promotes healing of skin wounds.
- Soothes skin irritations.
- Relieves ulcers.

HOW TO USE IT
Use prepared ointment or extract on skin wounds, insect bites, chafing, or other irritations.

Personal Advice

Some comfrey salves on the market specifically recommend use by nursing mothers with chafed nipples. However, since comfrey should not be ingested by infants, I would advise against this use.

CORDYCEPS
• *Cordyceps sinensis* •

FACTS

An extract derived from this Chinese mushroom or fungus has become a favorite of the gym crowd, who are constantly on the lookout for natural substances that will enhance endurance and stamina. Cordyceps became well known in 1993 when China's Olympic athletes attributed their winning performances to using it daily. Although cordyceps sounds unappetizing—it grows on dead insects or caterpillars—it was so highly prized by the ancient Chinese that it was used exclusively in the Emperor's palace. Traditional Chinese healers recommend cordyceps to increase energy, improve lung capacity, and as an overall tonic, similar to ginseng. Animal studies have shown that this herb will make mice swim for longer periods of time before succumbing to exhaustion than untreated mice. Athletes who use cordyceps claim that it enables them to work out harder and recover faster. It is also reputed to enhance sexual performance in men. Cordyceps appears to help the body better cope with stress, which could explain why it works well for competitive athletes.

POSSIBLE BENEFITS
- Improves physical endurance.
- Fortifies the body against stress.

HOW TO USE IT
Take 1 to 3 capsules or 1 to 2 drops of extract in liquid before a workout.

CRANBERRY
• *Vaccinium macrocarpon* •

FACTS

Americans eat about 117 million pounds of cranberry sauce each year, most of it during November and December. But don't wait for Thanksgiving! The common cranberry is one of nature's best weapons against cystitis and urinary tract infections. For years, doctors have routinely advised patients to drink cranberry juice to prevent urinary infections. In fact, it is cited as an effective remedy for this problem in the *U.S. Pharmacopeia*, the official listing of drugs in the United States. At one time, scientists believed that cranberry acidified the urine and, in the process, killed invading bacteria that could cause infection. Recently, however, Dr. Anthony Sabota, a scientist at Youngstown State University in Ohio, offered another possible explanation. His studies suggest that cranberry prevents bacteria from sticking to the wall of the bladder, thus flushing the potential troublemakers out of the body before they can do their damage. A 1994 study published in the *Journal of the American Medical Association* showed that older women who regularly drank cranberry juice cocktail—the kind sold in supermarkets—had a significantly lower rate of bacteria and pus in their urine, which increases the risk of infection, than women who drank a similar drink without cranberry juice. Similar to blueberries and bilberries, cranberry contains anthocyanidins, natural antibiotics. Cranberries (along with strawberries and grapes) contain *ellagic acid,* a natural antioxidant that blocks the effects of damaging free radicals. Native Americans used the whole dried cranberries to help disinfect wounds. Unfortunately, commercially prepared cranberry juice beverages are often laden with sugar and calories. Capsules of cranberry extract available in health food stores are not only more potent but less caloric.

POSSIBLE BENEFITS
- Prevents the spread of bacterial infection in the urinary tract.

HOW TO USE IT
Take up to 3 capsules daily.

CAUTION: If you suspect that you have a urinary tract infection, see your doctor at once. Untreated, it can lead to serious complications.

Personal Advice
Although they may provide adequate protection against infection, the cranberry juice cocktails sold in grocery stores are highly sweetened and processed. This is definitely not the kind of juice I advise people to use. Look for unsweetened, unprocessed products in specialty food stores or health food stores. Real cranberry juice is very tart, but also very effective. Some health food stores carry a natural, unprocessed cranberry juice–apple juice combination beverage, which is okay to use as long as it contains no added sugar.

DANDELION
....
• *Taraxacum officinale* •

FACTS

Dandelion is a natural diuretic and digestive aid. Its high mineral content may help prevent iron-deficiency anemia. This herb also reduces high blood pressure, probably due to its diuretic action. Dandelion is rich in *potassium*, which works with sodium to regulate the body's water balance and normalize heart rhythms. This vital mineral is often flushed from the body by synthetic diuretics. Dandelion enhances liver and gallbladder function, and has traditionally been used by herbal healers to treat liver disorders, such as jaundice. Dandelion is rich in *lecithin*, a substance researchers believe may protect against cirrhosis of the liver. It is also a wonderful source of carotenoids, which are converted into vitamin A in the body. In fact, it has more carotenoids than carrots!

POSSIBLE BENEFITS
- Helps rid body of excess water and salt.
- May decrease high blood pressure by ridding the body of excess fluid, thus reducing the amount of fluid the heart must pump to circulate blood.
- Good for the digestion.
- Protects against liver and gallbladder disorders.
- May protect against iron-deficiency anemia.

HOW TO USE IT
Take up to 3 capsules daily.
Mix 10 to 30 drops extract in juice or water daily.

Personal Advice
A combination of dandelion root, ginseng, and ginger root has worked wonders for people suffering from low blood sugar in conjunction with

a sound nutritional diet. A cup of this special blend using either the extracts or dried herbs 3 times a day will do the trick.

CAUTION: Do not take dandelion or any other diuretic herb in combination with diuretic medicines like Lasix or hydrochlorothiazide.

DEVIL'S CLAW

• *Harpagophytum procumbens* •

FACTS

The root of this herb has been popular in Africa and Europe for more than 250 years, but it is just being discovered in the United States. Devil's claw is primarily used as an anti-inflammatory and as a painkiller for arthritis and rheumatism. Recent studies done in France and Germany compare its anti-inflammatory action to the drugs cortisone and phenylbutazone.

POSSIBLE BENEFITS
   • Promotes flexibility in the joints, reducing the pain of
      arthritis and rheumatism.

HOW TO USE IT
   Take up to 3 capsules daily.

CAUTION: Do not use during pregnancy.

DONG QUAI

• *Angelica sinensis* •

FACTS

Dubbed the *female ginseng,* dong quai is an all-purpose herb for a wide range of female gynecological problems. For centuries, Chinese women have used this herb to regulate the menstrual cycle and quell painful menstrual cramps caused by uterine contractions. Modern herbalists use dong quai to eliminate the discomfort of premenstrual syndrome and to help women resume normal menstruation after going off the birth-control pill. Researchers have discovered that dong quai contains antispasmodic compounds that can relax smooth muscle tissue. This could explain its purported effectiveness as a treatment for menstrual cramps. For centuries, Asian healers have used dong quai as a cure for hot flashes and other symptoms of menopause caused by hormonal changes. In fact, it had been assumed that dong quai had estrogenic activity, and could be used instead of conventional hormone-replacement therapy. However, a recent clinical study, conducted by Kaiser Permanente Medical Care in Oakland, California, on the effect of dong quai in the treatment of menopausal symptoms, had disappointing results. In the twelve-week study involving seventy-one women, about half took 4.5 grams of dried root daily while the other half took a placebo. Both groups of women experienced a decline in symptoms, but the dong quai takers did not fare appreciably better than the placebo takers. Critics of the study contend that it was not accurate because dong quai is not meant to work alone, but in conjunction with up to ten different herbs. The study did not investigate whether dong quai is useful in treating menstrual cramps.

Rich in vitamins and minerals, including A, B, and E, this herb may prevent anemia. Dong quai has also been used to treat insomnia and high blood pressure for both sexes. Both men and women use this herb as a blood tonic. It is one of the most widely used herbs in Asia; dong quai duck is a popular Cantonese dish.

POSSIBLE BENEFITS

- Overall tonic for female reproductive system.
- Reduces menstrual cramping.
- Reduces PMS.
- May relieve symptoms of menopause with other herbs.
- Prevents anemia.
- Lowers high blood pressure.

HOW TO USE IT

Take up to 3 capsules daily.

CAUTION: Do not use during pregnancy, or if you are still menstruating and typically have a heavy flow. Dong quai may cause photosensitivity, which means that it increases the risk of getting a sunburn; therefore, while taking this herb, stay out of the sun as much as possible and always wear sunscreen on exposed areas.

ECHINACEA
• *Echinacea angustifolia* •

FACTS

In the first edition of the *Herb Bible,* I noted that echinacea, a popular herb at the turn of the century, was beginning to attract the attention of physicians and scientists because of its ability to boost immune function. In less than a decade, echinacea has become the top-selling herb in the United States. When it comes to tackling a cold or mild infection, there is no better treatment. A recent placebo-controlled double-blind study conducted in Sweden showed that echinacea can reduce at least twelve clinical symptoms of bad colds. Patients who took echinacea suffered less severe respiratory symptoms and got well faster than those who did not. Even better, there were no side effects. The best way to take echinacea is at the first sign of a cold or viral infection. Contrary to popular opinion, echinacea does not help to prevent colds and should not be taken daily. Rather, save it for when you really need an immune boost!

We owe Native Americans a debt of gratitude for introducing the settlers to the wonders of this purple-cone-flower plant. Indians of the Great Plains first used this herb as a remedy for snakebites and other skin wounds. They also applied the root of this plant directly to the mouth for toothaches and sore throats. Word of echinacea's healing properties traveled back to Europe, where it has become one of the most sought-after herbs and one of the better researched as well. Many studies have shown that echinacea prevents the formation of an enzyme called *hyaluronidase,* which destroys a natural barrier between healthy tissue and unwanted pathogenic organisms. Thus, echinacea helps the body maintain its line of defense against unwanted invaders, especially viruses. In 1972, a study appeared in the *Journal of Medical Chemistry,* showing that an echinacea extract inhibited tumor growth in rats. Echinacea has also been used to help restore normal immune function in patients receiving chemotherapy. In 1978, a study in *Planta Medica* showed that a root extract destroyed both herpes and influenza viruses.

Echinacea has also been used successfully to treat *candida,* an annoying and persistent fungal infection. In fact, patients treated with an antifungal cream and echinacea extract were less likely to suffer a recurrence than those treated solely with the antifungal cream.

POSSIBLE BENEFITS
- Boosts the immune system.
- Promotes healing of skin wounds.
- Fights bacterial and viral infections.
- Shortens the duration of colds and flu.

HOW TO USE IT
Take up to 240 mg. of echinacea capsules or tablets daily. I take a combination of echinacea and American feverfew in tablet form at the first sign of a cold

or flu. To ward off infection, I take 5 tablets daily for up to 3 days. It seems to do the trick.

Mix 15 to 30 drops extract in liquid every 3 hours.

Personal Advice

Many of the active compounds in echinacea can be destroyed during processing. Freeze-drying is the most effective way to preserve this herb's healing properties. A fully potent echinacea extract will create a tingling sensation on the tongue. If yours doesn't, you're missing out on some important compounds.

> **CAUTION:** Since echinacea stimulates immune function, I don't recommend it for people with autoimmune diseases, such as rheumatoid arthritis or lupus. Echinacea is wonderful for mild infections, but if you have a severe infection—if your fever persists for more than 24 hours, or if your respiratory symptoms do not abate within a few days—call your doctor.

ELDERBERRY

• *Sambuccua canadensis nigra* •

FACTS

For centuries, the berry from the elderberry tree has been a popular Gypsy remedy for colds, influenza, and neuralgia. Finally, there is solid scientific evidence to back up the folklore, thanks to Israeli researcher Dr. Madeliene Mumcuoglu, Ph.D., of Hadassah-Hebrew University Medical Center. In 1980, Dr. Mumcuoglu, intrigued by elderberry's reputation as a cure for colds and flu, did her thesis on the antiviral effects of elderberry. She patented a procedure to isolate the potent disease-fighting compounds from elderberry, then tested her extract on patients with flu. In a double-blind study, patients were given either elderberry extract or a placebo. Within twenty-four hours, 20 percent of those patients taking the extract had a dramatic improvement in symptoms such as muscle aches, fevers and coughing. By the second day, 73 percent showed improvement and, by the third day, 90 percent showed improvement. In the group not taking elderberry, only 16 percent had a reduction in symptoms by day two. How does elderberry fight the flu? Compounds in elderberry bind with viruses before they can penetrate the walls of cells, thereby inhibiting their ability to spread. Since elderberry is nontoxic, it is safe even for children.

The hot tea promotes sweating and is soothing for upper-respiratory infections. Externally, it has been used to relieve skin inflammation, such as eczema. In ancient times, elderberry trees were believed to have special mystical properties, and it was considered good luck to plant a tree near your house to protect against disease and evil spirits. There is even one planted outside of Westminster Abbey for this purpose. Elderberries are also a good source of vitamins A, B, and C. Cooked berries can be used in pies and jams.

POSSIBLE BENEFITS
- Relieves symptoms of coughs and colds.
- Applied externally, useful for burns, rashes, and minor skin problems.

HOW TO USE IT
For children over thirteen and adults: Take 4 tablespoons of elderberry extract or lozenges daily. For ages one to twelve, give 2 to 3 tablespoons daily.

A liquid made of elderberry juice boiled together with crabapple and a little sugar to form a syrup is an old Gypsy remedy for coughs and bronchial infections, but store-bought elderberry tea and honey will also do the trick.

CAUTION: The seeds from the raw elderberry plant are toxic; therefore, don't eat the berry unless it is cooked. Store-bought elderberry preparations are perfectly safe.

The Legend of the Elder

The elder tree was reputed to be the favorite tree of witches, who supposedly resided in its branches. In the Middle Ages, nearly everyone knew that cutting down an elder tree would incur the wrath of the witches who called it home. There were many tales of angry witches taking vengeance on babies whose unwitting parents put them in a cradle of elder wood.

EPHEDRA

• *Ephedra sinica* •

FACTS

Known as *ma huang* in China, where it is grown in the Inner Mongolia region, this herb has been used for more than four thousand years to treat asthma and upper respiratory infections. Ephedra, which is cultivated in the dry regions of North America, contains two alkaloids, *ephedrine* and *pseudoephedrine,* which today are used in many over-the-counter cold and allergy medications. Ephedrine is used in weight-loss products because it suppresses appetite while turning up metabolism. Products containing high doses of ephredine have been promoted as "natural highs," but these products are dangerous and should not be used. In fact, there have been deaths linked to the abuse of ephedrine, resulting in the ban of ephedrine products in states such as Florida and New York. The FDA cautions against taking more than 24 mg. of ephedrine in a twenty-four-hour period and for more than seven days. Excessive intake of ephedra can increase blood pressure and place an unhealthy burden on the heart. It is particularly bad for people with heart conditions. However, if used correctly and conservatively, the natural herb ephedra is safe for most people and has been used successfully for thousands of years. In other words, a cup or two of ephedra tea is fine if you have a cold. Abusing ephedra, as with any other drug, is foolish.

Also called *Mormon tea* and *Squaw tea,* American ephedra was discovered by the early pioneers and Mormon settlers, who used it to treat asthma. It is also useful for headaches, fevers, and hay fever.

POSSIBLE BENEFITS
- Decongestant can relieve stuffy nose, watery eyes, and other cold and allergy symptoms.
- May help relieve headaches.
- Long-acting stimulant that can last up to 24 hours.
- Turns up metabolism.

HOW TO USE IT
Drink 1 cup ephedra tea to relieve cold or allergy symptoms. Do not use for more than seven days. Avoid drinking tea at night since it may keep you up.
Take up to 2 capsules daily; do not exceed 24 mg. daily. Do not take for more than 1 week.

CAUTION: Do not use this herb if you have high blood pressure, heart disease, diabetes, or thyroid disease except under the supervision of your doctor. Do not exceed recommended dose. If you are pregnant or nursing, check with your doctor before using any ephedra preparations.

EVENING PRIMROSE

• *Oenothera biennis* •

FACTS

Evening primrose is an American herb that was brought to Europe in the seventeenth century. Once called *king's cure-all,* this herb has been used for a wide range of problems. Native Americans used it as a painkiller and asthma treatment.

Evening primrose oil is a highly effective treatment for *polycystic breast disease,* a serious sounding name for a benign condition—cystic breasts. Women say that evening primrose oil relieves the pain and tenderness associated with this condition. It works especially well when combined with 400 IU of vitamin E daily.

Recently, *gamma linoleic acid* (GLA), a fatty acid found in evening primrose oil, has been used successfully as a treatment for rheumatoid arthritis. In one double-blind study involving fifty-six men and women with RA, one-half took GLA capsules or a sunflower oil placebo in addition to their regular medication. After six months, those taking GLA experienced a significant improvement in swelling, joint pain, and stiffness. Some were able to reduce the dose of their prescription medication. People taking sunflower capsules either stayed the same or worsened. For the second six months of the study, all patients were given GLA. At the end of a year, 50 per-cent of all patients showed significant improvement. Since RA is a degenerative condition that is difficult to treat, these findings are extremely impressive.

Studies have shown that evening primrose oil can help lower blood cholesterol. In fact, according to one Canadian study, patients who took 4 grams of Efamol, a brand of evening primrose oil, daily experienced a 31.5 percent decline in cholesterol after three months of treatment. Other studies have shown that evening primrose oil also reduces blood pressure. This herb is an old-time remedy for infantile eczema, or *cradle cap.* A 1987 study in the *British Journal of Dermatology* concluded that patients with eczema showed significant improvement after being treated with evening primrose oil and were able to reduce their dependence on steroids.

POSSIBLE BENEFITS
- Relieves symptoms of rheumatoid arthritis.
- Treatment for premenstrual breast pain and polycystic breasts.
- Reduces anxiety.
- Helps prevent heart disease and stroke by controlling high blood pressure and reducing cholesterol.
- Helps maintain healthy skin.

HOW TO USE IT
Take up to three 250 mg. capsules daily.

CAUTION: Patients taking phenothiazine drugs should not use evening primrose oil except under a doctor's supervision.

EYEBRIGHT
• *Euphrasia officinalis* •

FACTS

Since the Middle Ages, eyebright has been used as a tonic and an astringent. It is especially useful for eyestrain, eye inflammations, and other eye ailments. It can greatly relieve runny, sore, itchy eyes due to colds or allergies.

POSSIBLE BENEFITS
- An eyewash made of eyebright and other herbs can be soothing to irritated and inflamed eyes.
- Taken internally, it may help maintain good vision and eye health.

HOW TO USE IT

Take one capsule up to 3 times daily.

Mix 15 to 40 drops of extract in liquid every 3 to 4 hours.

Eyewash products containing euphrasia, plus other herbs such as goldenseal, bayberry, and raspberry leaves, are available commercially. Put eyewash in eyecup and rinse out eye 3 to 4 times daily.

Personal Advice

Hay-fever sufferers should try taking this herb for allergic eyes.

FENNEL

• *Foeniculum vulgare* •

FACTS

Fennel is one of those spices in your kitchen cabinet that can be put to many uses. For centuries, this herb has been used to relieve gas and to stimulate appetite. Fennel oil with honey in warm water is an old-time cough remedy that was used long before the arrival of the over-the-counter "ussins." Used externally, the oil is a folk remedy for joint inflammation caused by rheumatism and arthritis.

POSSIBLE BENEFITS

• Digestive aid that can relieve cramps and gas.
• Good expectorant for coughs and colds.
• Can improve a sluggish appetite.
• Relieves stiff, painful joints.

HOW TO USE IT

Mix 10 to 20 drops extract in water. Use warm water and a teaspoon of honey for a soothing drink daily.

The oil can be rubbed on affected parts of the body as needed to alleviate the pain of arthritis.

FENUGREEK

• *Trigonella graecum* •

FACTS

One of the oldest known medicinal plants, use of fenugreek dates back to the ancient Egyptians and Hippocrates. A popular folk remedy for sore throats and colds, this herb is also reputed to be an aphrodisiac. Fenugreek may also be useful against diabetes. In a study done in India involving insulin-dependent diabetics on low doses of insulin, pulverized seeds of fenugreek were shown to reduce blood sugar and harmful fats. The authors of the study suggested that diabetics may benefit by adding fenugreek seeds to their diets. Used externally, pulverized fenugreek seeds may help soothe skin irritations and reduce the pain of neuralgia, swollen glands, and tumors.

POSSIBLE BENEFITS
- Good expectorant for coughs and colds.
- As a gargle, can relieve sore throat.
- Useful for skin irritations and other inflammations.
- Lowers blood sugar.

HOW TO USE IT
Take up to 3 capsules daily.

To make a gargle, mix 1 tablespoon pulverized seed in 8 ounces hot water. Let steep for 10 minutes. Strain. Gargle every 3 hours up to 3 times daily, to relieve sore throat.

The seeds can be pulverized and made into a poultice that can be applied to painful areas of the body. Mix enough pulverized seeds in 8 ounces warm water to make a thick paste. Apply directly to the affected areas daily.

FEVERFEW
....
• *Chrysanthemum parthenium* •

FACTS

Legend has it that this herb saved the life of someone who had the misfortune of falling from the Parthenon, the famous temple in ancient Greece. Since that time, herbalists have used feverfew for a wide variety of problems. As its name suggests, it was used to help bring down a fever. The Greek herbalist Dioscorides is believed to have used this herb to treat arthritis. In 1649, Culpeper recommended it for women as a "general strengthener of their wombs," and also noted that "it is very effectual for all pains in the head." In 1772, John Hill, another famous herbalist, wrote that "in the worst headache, this herb exceeds whatever else is known."

Feverfew was all but forgotten until 1978, when British newspapers told of a woman who had cured her migraines with feverfew leaves. The articles caught the attention of serious medical researchers who decided to further examine this phenomenon. In 1985, the well-respected British medical journal *Lancet* reported that extracts of feverfew inhibited the release of two inflammatory substances—*serotonin,* from platelets and *prostaglandin,* from white blood cells—both thought to contribute to the onset of migraine attacks and perhaps even to play a role in rheumatoid arthritis. In 1988, *Lancet* also reported that a carefully designed study proved what herbalists have known for centuries: Feverfew can help prevent migraine headaches or lessen their severity. The primary active ingredient in feverfew is *parthenolide,* which inhibits the release of chemicals in the body that can cause inflammation. It also decreases the secretion of *serotonin* and *histamine,* two naturally occurring chemicals within the body that, if not tightly controlled, can trigger headaches and other problems. Because of its anti-inflammatory action, feverfew is under investigation as a treatment for rheumatoid arthritis.

POSSIBLE BENEFITS

- May be of great help to migraine sufferers, reducing the number of headaches.

May reduce severity of migraine symptoms, including nausea, vomiting, and head pain.

HOW TO USE IT

Take one 125 mg. capsule daily standardized to .2 percent parthenolide.

Personal Advice

It may take several months before migraine sufferers notice an improvement, but it is well worth the wait. It seems to work well for most people as a preventive in migraine headaches. Some herbalists suggest taking an additional dose if you feel a migraine coming on.

CAUTION: Feverfew can interfere with blood clotting; therefore, if you are taking any anticoagulants, you must be closely monitored by your physician if you are also taking feverfew. Feverfew should not be used during pregnancy or by nursing mothers. Chewing the whole leaf can cause mouth ulcers.

FO-TI

• Polygonum multiforum •

FACTS

Known as *ho shou wu* in China, this herb is used primarily as a rejuvenating tonic. The Chinese claim that fo-ti can prevent hair from going gray, as well as preventing other signs of premature aging. It is also believed to increase fertility and maintain strength and vigor. Animal tests using fo-ti extract show antitumor activity. This herb also appears to protect against heart disease by preventing blood clots and reducing blood pressure.

POSSIBLE BENEFITS

- May help slow signs of premature aging.
- Used generally as a tonic to maintain health and energy.
- Good for heart health.
- May help prevent cancer.

HOW TO USE IT

Take up to 3 capsules daily.

GARCINIA CAMBOGIA

• *Garcinia cambogia* •

FACTS

Known as *Malabar tamarind,* this member of the citrus family produces a tropical fruit that is used in Indian cooking—especially in curries—and as a preservative. Several species of the Garcinia family have been used for centuries in Ayurvedic medicine to treat a wide range of ailments from arthritis to spongy gums and, more interestingly, as a natural appetite suppressant. Only during the past few decades have scientists begun to take a more serious look at traditional medicine systems and, in particular, have subjected folk medicines to rigorous laboratory testing. The results were often surprising. In 1965, scientists discovered that the principle active ingredient in Garcinia cambogia was hydrocitric acid (H.C.A.). In 1977, scientists reported in the *American Journal of Clinical Nutrition* that hydrocitric acid burned fat but did not cause the loss of body protein or lean mass in obese animals. Within a decade, human studies confirmed that H.C.A. could help promote modest weight loss in obese people. H.C.A. appears to work by temporarily blocking the synthesis of fat, so that the body is forced to burn more calories. Word soon spread about this amazing fat burner and, by the mid-1990s, products containing H.C.A. were all the rage. Today you can find Garcinia cambogia (or H.A.) in numerous weight-loss products, diet drinks, and diet bars. However, the *Journal of the American Medical Association* reported that garcinia was no better than a placebo in a recent study performed at the Obesity Research Center at St. Luke's-Roosevelt Hospital in New York. In the study, 135 overweight people were given either garcinia or a placebo supplement daily for twelve weeks. At the end of the study, the garcinia group did not fare any better than the placebo group in terms of weight loss or fat mass loss.

In my experience, garcinia may work for some but not all people. Successful weight loss depends on many factors, especially eating the right foods in the right amounts, and burning calories through exercise. Alas, when it comes to permanent weight loss, there is no magic bullet.

An added bonus: H.C.A. can lower high triglyceride levels, a condition which increases the risk of heart attack and stroke.

POSSIBLE BENEFITS

- Reputed but not proven to promote the burning of calories and prevent the storage of fat.
- May suppress appetite.

HOW TO USE IT

Take 1 tablet with a fatty meal. Drink at least 8 glasses water daily.

CAUTION: This supplement should not be used by pregnant or lactating women.

GARLIC

• *Allium sativum* •

FACTS

Garlic may be the wonder drug of the herbal world. The ancient Egyptians not only worshipped garlic but fed it to their slaves to keep them healthy, for good reason. This amazing herb does everything from aid in the treatment of ear infections to help prevent heart disease and cancer. It has even been used to treat tuberculosis, with good results. Biologist Louis Pasteur put garlic to the test by putting a few cloves in a petri dish full of bacteria. Much to his surprise, he discovered that garlic could indeed kill troublesome microorganisms.

In the 1950s, Dr. Albert Schweitzer used garlic to treat cholera, typhus, and amebic dysentery while working as a missionary in Africa. During both world wars, before the widespread availability of antibiotics, garlic was used on the battlefield to disinfect wounds and prevent gangrene. In fact, the Soviet army relied so heavily on garlic that it earned the name "Russian penicillin."

Garlic is also used as an anticoagulant to resolve fresh blood clots and some, but not all, studies have shown that it can lower cholesterol while increasing the level of beneficial HDLs, the so-called good cholesterol. Not all commercial garlic preparations can lower cholesterol, however. Be sure to use those with *allicin,* the primary cholesterol-lowering ingredient. (Allicin is missing from steam-distilled garlic oil.) Garlic also lowers blood pressure. In fact, according to a study published in *Atherosclerosis,* when patients with hyperlipoproteinemia ate garlic, blood pressure declined along with levels of LDL (low-density lipoprotein) and fibrinogen. An added bonus was that anticlotting factor levels increased, reducing the risk of blood clots.

There is evidence that garlic can affect the mortality rate of heart attack victims. Researcher Arun Noria at Tagore Medical College in Udaipur, India, monitored 432 heart attack survivors for three years. Half the group drank the juice of six to ten garlic cloves each day. The other half drank a garlic-scented placebo. The garlic eaters experienced 32 percent fewer recurrent heart attacks, and 45 percent fewer deaths.

Hippocrates is believed to have used garlic to treat uterine cancer. We now know that garlic is toxic to some tumor cells; it is being investigated by the National Cancer Institute for its cancer-inhibiting properties. According to a recent NCI study of four thousand people from Italy and China, those who recalled eating diets high in garlic and other alliums, including onions, had a substantially lower incidence of stomach cancer than those who abstained from this pungent herb. Recently, researchers from Memorial Sloan Kettering Cancer Center in New York found that a compound found in aged garlic dramatically slows down the growth of human prostate cancer cells in the test tube. They are hopeful that garlic may prove to be a useful treatment for prostate cancer.

Garlic oil can relieve earaches and can help heal minor skin disorders. On top of everything else, garlic is good for indigestion.

POSSIBLE BENEFITS
- Helps prevent heart disease by reducing blood pressure and blood lipids.
- Helps fight infection.
- Can destroy some types of cancer cells.
- Excellent digestive aid.

HOW TO USE IT
Aged, odorless garlic is the preferred capsule form. Take 1 capsule up to 3 times daily. Parsley seed oil can be used in a capsule along with extract of garlic to eliminate the breath-odor problem.

Stir-frying the cloves for a few minutes will help eliminate garlic breath and aftertaste. Two to three cooked cloves daily will give maximum benefits.

Put a few drops of warm garlic oil in the ear canal for earache. Cover with cotton and leave in for an hour.

For sprains, aches, and minor skin disorders, rub it directly on affected areas several times daily.

CAUTION: Since garlic is a natural blood thinner, there is a slim chance that it may interact with anticoagulant medication, such as coumadin. If you are taking blood thinners and using garlic, be vigilant about having your blood monitored. Garlic should not be used by women who are breast-feeding, because it can pass to the breast milk and cause colic in infants.

GINGER

• *Zingiber officinale* •

FACTS

Remember when your mother used to give you ginger ale when you felt nauseated? She knew what she was doing. Ginger is a time-proven remedy for upset stomach, indigestion, and cramps. The Chinese have been using ginger for more than two thousand years.

Ginger is a natural anti-inflammatory. Recent studies have documented another use for ginger—as a treatment for arthritis. Studies show that patients who ate lightly cooked fresh ginger or took a standardized ginger supplement showed improvement in swelling, morning stiffness, pain, and joint mobility. I have recommended a standardized ginger extract to many people with arthritis, with excellent results. Ginger is also a wonderful treatment for motion sickness and, in many cases, may work better than standard drugs. If you suffer from motion sickness, take ginger capsules about 30 minutes prior to engaging in an activity that triggers this problem.

The Japanese serve pickled ginger slices between sushi courses to clear the palate and aid digestion. Grated ginger combined with olive oil is an old-fashioned but quite effective remedy for dandruff. Apply to scalp before you shampoo. A few drops of this oil can also be warmed and used in the ear to soothe earaches.

POSSIBLE BENEFITS
- Reduces arthritis symptoms.
- Calms an upset stomach.
- Relieves motion sickness.
- Eases cold symptoms.

HOW TO USE IT

Take up to three capsules daily to relieve symptoms as
needed. It is safe to take up to 2000 mg. or even
more ginger daily. (I take a nutraceutical herbal extract [EV EXT 77™], which is a combination of a
unique subspecies of this plant, for joint pain twice
daily with food.) Ginger tea can be found at most
natural food stores.

Mix 15 drops of extract in warm water. This drink can
be taken up to 3 times daily. For external use, mix
15 drops extract in 1 cup warm vegetable oil. Mash
fresh ginger, soak in cotton ball, and apply juice directly to inflamed area.

Personal Advice

I was discussing certain herbs on a Los Angeles talk show when the host
complained that the early-morning drive to the studio, down the steep,
winding roads of the Hollywood Hills left him feeling nauseated. I suggested that he try gingerroot capsules. It worked. The next day he spent
a full five minutes on the show talking about the wonders of this "newfound" remedy for motion sickness!

Ginger is a natural blood thinner, which is good, because it can
prevent the formation of potentially dangerous blood clots. If you are
taking other prescription blood thinners, however, be sure that your
blood is routinely monitored.

CAUTION: In moderate amounts, ginger is a safe remedy for *morning sickness,* a common condition suffered by half of all pregnant women. There is a theoretical risk that excessive ginger intake can promote spontaneous abortion. In fact, Chinese herbalists caution against gorging on ginger during the first months of pregnancy. However, there have not been any documented cases of women losing pregnancies due to ginger intake. To be on the safe side, however, use this herb judiciously during pregnancy—do not exceed 2000 mg. daily. Other commercial antinauseants should not be used during pregnancy because of the possibility that they may cross the placenta and adversely affect the fetus.

GINKGO
• *Ginkgo biloba* •

FACTS

For more than five thousand years, Chinese herbalists have recommended this ancient remedy for coughs, asthma, and inflammations due to allergies. Although the ginkgo tree dates back more than two hundred million years—some live as long as four thousand years—we are just beginning to understand its medicinal value. Ginkgo is one of the most well-researched herbs in the world. Most of the research is being done in France and other European countries, where ginkgo is the number-one prescribed drug. Ginkgo is rich in flavonoids, antioxidant compounds found in plants that protect against heart disease, cancer, and premature aging. It also contains biologically active compounds called *terpenoids,* which include gingolides and bilobalide.

Ginkgo exerts a positive effect on the vascular system, the body's vast network of blood vessels, which delivers blood and oxygen to various organ systems. Similar to pine-bark extract (see page 132) ginkgo helps regulate *nitric oxide,* a free radical produced in the body that, among other things, controls the muscular tone of blood vessels. Too much nitric oxide can hamper circulation. Ginkgo is best known as a brain booster, for good reason. Ginkgo has been shown to improve memory and to relieve signs of senility, probably due to the increased blood flow to the brain. Recently, ginkgo extract was tested at the New York Institute for Medical Research on patients suffering from dementia, caused either by Alzheimer's disease or stroke. In the study, 327 patients were given either 120 mg. of ginkgo extract daily or a placebo. Out of the 137 patients who completed the study, 30 percent of those taking ginkgo performed better on tests measuring reasoning ability and memory than the placebo takers. Although researchers said the gingko effect was modest, they were nonetheless excited by the results, because few drugs have been shown to have any positive impact on dementia. It is quite possible that taking ginkgo long before age-related brain problems might arise can help prevent these problems in the first place.

Ginkgo is also being touted as a sexual revitalizer for men. In one study reported in the *Journal of Urology,* fifty impotent men were given 240 mg. of ginkgo extract daily for nine months. Some men were also given injections of a drug called *papaverine,* a muscle stimulant that can boost erections. Within eight weeks, the ginkgo supplement alone greatly improved erections in both groups of men. Although Viagra is now being touted as the drug of choice for potency problems, it is not suitable for many men, particularly those taking certain heart medications. Ginkgo may be a safe alternative for these men if used under a doctor's supervision.

Ginkgo also helps prevent blood clots and has been used quite successfully for problems related to poor circulation, such as *phlebitis* (inflammation of a vein) and *diabetic peripheral vascular disease,* caused by poor circulation. In Europe, ginkgo has been used to treat *tinnitus* (ringing in the ears), vertigo, and hearing problems.

In 1988, Dr. Elias J. Corey, professor of chemistry at Harvard University, synthesized a ginkgo compound called *ginkgolide B,* thus increasing the commercial possibilities for this herb in the United States. Among other things, ginkgolide B is being investigated in the prevention of the rejection of transplanted organs. Researchers are hopeful that it may one day spawn new drugs for asthma and toxic-shock syndrome.

POSSIBLE BENEFITS

- Improves circulation throughout the body.
- Improves mental functioning and the ability to concentrate.
- May be useful to relieve symptoms of Alzheimer's disease.
- Successfully used to treat hemorrhoids.

HOW TO USE IT

Take 60 mg. capsules or tablets 2 to 3 times daily. Look for standardized products containing gingko-leaf extracts (24 percent flavonoids and 6 percent terpenoids or terpene). I take a combination standardized ginkgo biloba extract with club moss, phosphatidyl choline, inositol, and serine twice daily to keep my memory and concentration strong.

Personal Advice

Long-term use is believed to be safe. No known serious side effects have been reported.

ASIAN GINSENG

• *Panax ginseng* •

FACTS

Ginseng is best known as the herb to boost energy. It is used to reduce stress, speed recovery from illness, and improve physical and mental stamina. Similar to other tonic herbs, ginseng is not regarded as a medical treatment but, rather, as the ultimate herb to enhance wellness. Indeed, the reverence in which some hold ginseng is reflected in its botanical name *panax,* which is derived from the Greek word for *panacea.*

Ginseng, or *ren shen* in Mandarin, literally means "root of man," so named because the root of this plant resembles the shape of a human body. For the past two decades, ginseng has been touted as a wonder herb. Many athletes swear that it gives them the competitive edge and, while studies have shown that ginseng enhances physical performance in animals, its effects on humans in this regard have not been widely studied. Recent studies involving 500 people taking ginseng along with other vitamins and minerals noted that participants felt they had experienced an improved quality of life. Obviously, anything that boosts energy and improves general well-being is going to have a positive effect on your outlook.

Rich in natural estrogenlike compounds, ginseng is used to alleviate hot flashes and some of the more unpleasant signs of menopause.

Although we may credit ourselves with discovering this herb, in reality, the Chinese have been using it for more than five thousand years! Ginseng was mentioned in the *Shen Nong Herbal* compiled between the first and second centuries, as a "superior drug" suitable for long-term use without toxic effects. The Chinese were referring to *panax ginseng,* a variety grown in China. Today, there are three different herbs that fall under the label *ginseng.* In addition to panax, American ginseng or *Panax quinquefolius* (see page 94) is very popular in China. What is called *Siberian ginseng* or *Eleutherococcus senticosus* (see page 95) is technically not ginseng at all, but has many of the same properties of ginseng and is, therefore, used the same way. Although all forms of ginseng have similar properties, there are some subtle differences.

Western interest in ginseng began in the 1960s, when researchers in China, the Soviet Union, Japan, and European countries began to take a serious look at this herb. In 1969, Soviet scientist I. I. Brekhman, Ph.D., reported that Soviet soldiers who took ginseng extract were able to run faster in a 3-kilometer race than another group given a placebo. Dr. Brekhman was the first to call ginseng an *adaptogen,* which he described as, basically, any substance that enables the body to better cope with stress. According to Dr. Brekhman, an adaptogen has the unique ability to normalize body functions. For instance, if blood-sugar levels drop too low, or if blood pressure climbs too high, an adaptogen will bring the body back to normal levels. In his writings, Dr. Brekhman has noted that adaptogens work best on people who are neither in peak condition nor in poor health. Rather, they appear to do the most for people who fall somewhere between those two extremes.

Studies in Japan showed that mice who were fed ginseng learned to perform tasks at a faster rate and made fewer mistakes. In the 1970s, Japanese researchers found that rats who were fed a high-cholesterol diet showed a drop in cholesterol, especially LDL, and a rise in beneficial HDL cholesterol after being given ginseng. A recent study at the Defense Institute of Physiology and Allied Sciences in Delhi, India, showed that rats given ginseng were better able to endure high altitudes and cold temperatures than control rats. Another study at Japan's Kanazawa University found that unpurified saponins from panax ginseng not only inhibited the growth of cancer cells but actually converted the diseased cells into normal cells. Undoubtedly, further studies will be done to determine if some form of ginseng can be used as a cancer treatment.

There have been very few studies of ginseng done in the United States. One famous negative report published in the *Journal of the American Medical Association* described the so-called ginseng abuse syndrome. The article said that heavy users of ginseng were subject to hypertension, nervousness, and insomnia, among other ills. The study, however, included people who took all forms of ginseng—root, powder, extract—as well as those who abused ginseng by injecting it into their veins. The article did not differentiate between caffeine users and noncaffeine users, caffeine being a substance that could cause similar effects. The article is considered by knowledgeable herbal researchers to be completely off base.

Long before ginseng was studied by the scientific community, Chinese healers were prescribing ginseng to normalize blood pressure, improve blood circulation, and prevent heart disease, among other things. For centuries, ginseng has been purported to be an aphrodisiac, although this claim has never been seriously studied. The main active ingredients in ginseng are called *ginsenosides*. The higher the quantity of ginsenosides, the better the quality of the ginseng.

POSSIBLE BENEFITS

- Increases physical and mental endurance.
- Helps the body adjust to stressful situations.

- Normalizes body functions.
- Reduces cholesterol.
- Increases energy.
- May help reduce discomfort caused by menopause.
- May inhibit growth of cancerous tumors.
- May enhance sexual desire.

HOW TO USE IT

Take up to 3 capsules daily between meals or on an
empty stomach. Look for standardized products of
at least 7 percent ginsenosides.
Drink 1 cup tea daily.
Mix 5 to 10 grams powder in liquid daily.

CAUTION: Some people may find panax ginseng too stimulating, especially if used before bedtime. Therefore, use early in the day. High doses may make you feel jittery. Do not exceed 5 to 10 grams daily. In very rare cases, some people may develop headaches or high blood pressure from panax ginseng. If you have high blood pressure, check with your doctor before using this product. Take ginseng 1 hour before or after eating. Vitamin C can interfere with the absorption of ginseng. If you take a vitamin C supplement, wait 2 hours before or after taking ginseng to do so. In rare cases, ginseng can cause vaginal bleeding in menopausal women, which isn't dangerous, but could be mistaken as a symptom of uterine cancer. If you experience any vaginal bleeding, however, be sure to notify your doctor, and be sure to tell him or her that you are taking ginseng. Pregnant women should not use ginseng.

Personal Advice

There are two types of ginseng—red and white—which reflect differences in the processing of the root. White ginseng is simply cleaned and dried; thus, it retains its natural white color. Red ginseng is steamed with a solution of herbs and is considered of superior quality. There have been many reports of diluted or adulterated ginseng products. Your best bet is to buy standardized, guaranteed-potency ginseng from a reputable company. In addition, keep in mind that the ginseng-flavored soft drinks sold in many health food stores do not offer any of the benefits of true ginseng. I take a combination of ten of the world's best known ginsengs all in one tablet! It is both easy and effective.

AMERICAN GINSENG
• *Panax quinquefolius* •

FACTS

You may think of Wisconsin as the cheese basket of the United States, but it is internationally known for another export—ginseng. In fact, Wisconsin-grown ginseng is highly valued throughout the Orient. Although it is very similar to panax ginseng, and offers many of the same benefits, Chinese herbalists believe that it is somewhat milder and perhaps less stimulating. They often prescribe American ginseng for times of acute stress, such as after a long illness. Native American Indians have used the root of this plant to relieve vomiting and nausea. Some tribes used it in their love potions. American colonists began using ginseng in the early 1700s. The Eclectics, nineteenth-century physicians who rejected synthetic drugs in favor of plant medicines, recommended American ginseng as a mild stimulant and aphrodisiac.

POSSIBLE BENEFITS
- Helps body adapt to stress.
- Normalizes body functions.
- Works as a mild stimulant.
- Enhances physical and mental performance.
- Reduces cholesterol.
- May inhibit growth of cancerous tumors.

HOW TO USE IT

Take 2 to 3 capsules daily on an empty stomach. Look
   for standardized products of at least 7 percent ginsenosides.

Mix 1 to 2 teaspoons powder in warm liquid daily.

Drink 1 cup tea daily.

SIBERIAN GINSENG

• *Eleutherococcus senticosus* •

FACTS

If Asian and American ginseng are first cousins in the plant world,
Siberian ginseng is a distant relative with a remarkable resemblance to
its famous kin. The active chemical ingredients are called *eleutherosides*.
Grown in Siberia, this herb is believed to relieve physical and mental
stress, and has been used to treat bronchitis and chronic lung ailments.
Similar to true ginseng, it normalizes blood pressure and reduces blood
cholesterol. Studies of Siberian ginseng by I. I. Brekhman show that,
like members of the panax family, it can increase stamina. In fact, Siberian ginseng is routinely used by Russian athletes.

POSSIBLE BENEFITS

- Helps body withstand stress.
- Improves mental alertness.
- Helps cure colds and infections.
- Improves overall health.
- Helps prevent heart disease by reducing cholesterol
    and blood pressure.

HOW TO USE IT

Take 2 to 3 capsules daily on an empty stomach.

Mix 5 to 10 drops extract in warm liquid daily.

Personal Advice

Chinese healers believe that Siberian ginseng is one of the best remedies for insomnia.

GOLDENSEAL

• *Hydrastis canadensis* •

FACTS

One of the oldest recorded remedies, goldenseal is a broad-spectrum herb that is growing in popularity. In fact, it has become so popular that herbalists are concerned that it will become extinct, and caution against overuse. Since there are other herbs (such as echinacea, elderberry, and olive-leaf extract) that can be used in place of goldenseal, for conservation purposes I suggest using these other herbs whenever possible, until the world's supply of goldenseal has been stabilized.

Discovered by the aborigines of northern Australia, goldenseal grows freely in the eastern United States and is being cultivated in the west. Long before antibiotics, preparations from this versatile plant were used as a treatment for gonorrhea and syphilis. Today, goldenseal is used to treat symptoms of colds and flu, as well as congestion due to inflammation of the mucous membranes. *Berberine,* an alkaloid in goldenseal, has mild antibiotic properties and is effective against protozoa such as giardia and trichomonas.

Goldenseal is also an excellent laxative, and can reduce irritation due to hemorrhoids. This herb is routinely used for female complaints, such as vaginitis. A douche of goldenseal can help relieve fungal infections, such as candida. Rubbed on the skin, goldenseal tea is a folk remedy for skin ailments including eczema, ringworm, and other inflammations. Used externally, it is an excellent antiseptic and can also soothe irritated gums and canker sores. Combined with myrrh, another Hot Hundred herb, goldenseal has been used to treat stomach ulcers.

POSSIBLE BENEFITS

- Anti-inflammatory action can soothe irritated mucous membranes.
- Relieves symptoms of colds and flu.
- Aids indigestion and constipation.
- Good for skin inflammations, such as eczema.
- Mouthwash can help prevent gum disease.
- Good douche for vaginal infections.
- Relieves discomfort caused by ulcers when used with myrrh.

HOW TO USE IT

Take 1 to 2 capsules up to 3 times daily for no more than two weeks.

Mix 5 to 10 drops in liquid up to 3 times daily.

Dissolve 1 teaspoon in 1 pint of hot water. Let stand until cool. Take 1 to 2 teaspoons 3 to 6 times daily.

For external use: Dissolve 1 tablespoon of powder in warm water. Let cool. Douche every 3 days for up to 2 weeks.

CAUTION: This herb can raise blood pressure, and should not be used by anyone with a history of high blood pressure. Do not use during pregnancy. Do not use for more than two weeks at a time. Eating the fresh plant can cause inflammation of the mucous tissue.

Gotu Kola
• *Centella Asiatica* •

FACTS

This herb was probably first used in India, where it is part of Ayurveda. It was also mentioned in the *Shennong Herbal.* In recent years, it has become popular in the West as a nerve tonic to promote relaxation and enhance memory. Indian healers used this herb to treat skin inflammations, and as a mild diuretic. Asian healers relied on gotu kola to treat emotional disorders, such as depression that may be rooted in physical problems. It has also been used to bring down a fever, and relieve congestion due to colds and upper-respiratory infections.

Recent studies show that gotu kola has a positive effect on the circulatory system: It seems to improve the flow of blood throughout the body by strengthening the veins and capillaries. It has been used successfully to treat phlebitis (inflammation of the veins), as well as leg cramps, swelling of the legs, and heaviness or tingling in the legs. It has been shown to be particularly useful for people who are inactive or confined to bed. Proponents of the herb also believe that its beneficial effect on circulation may help improve memory and brain function.

This herb also has an important role in gynecology. It has been used successfully to promote healing after episiotomy, a surgical incision of the vulva sometimes performed to prevent tearing during childbirth. In fact, in one study reported in a French medical journal in 1996, women treated with gotu kola after childbirth healed more rapidly than those given standard treatment.

POSSIBLE BENEFITS
- May help improve memory.
- Has a calming effect on the body.
- Good expectorant—can eliminate congestion due to colds.
- Promotes healing after childbirth.

- Improves circulation.
- Reduces pain and swelling due to phlebitis.

HOW TO USE IT

Take up to 3 capsules daily.
Mix 5 to 10 drops extract in liquid. Take 3 times daily.

CAUTION: Do not use during pregnancy. One manufacturer cautions that this herb should not be used by anyone with an overactive thyroid.

Loves Me—Loves Me Not

Before the days of Ouija boards, young women used the feathery seed balls of the dandelion to determine if their loves were really true. A maiden would blow on the dandelion three times. If at least one of the fuzzy seeds remained, it was taken as an omen that her sweetheart was thinking about her.

GRAPESEED EXTRACT

FACTS

A virtual unknown ten years ago, grapeseed extract has become one of the most popular herbs in the United States. Grapeseed extract contains antioxidant flavonoids called *proanthocyanidins,* which are also found in berries. Proanthycyanidins enhance the activity of vitamin C within the body. Grapeseed extract can prevent the oxidation of LDL, which leads to the formation of plaque or fatty deposits in the arteries. Grapeseed extract also helps to strengthen *capillaries,* the smallest blood vessels in the body, which are vulnerable to damage. Weakened capillaries can lead to easy bruising and varicose veins.

What's good for the heart often protects against cancer as well and, in this respect, when you take grapeseed extract you are killing two birds handily with one stone. Proanthocyanidins can block *free radicals* (unstable oxygen molecules found in the body) that are believed to be a leading cause of cancer. Grapeseed extract is also an anti-inflammatory, and has been used to treat arthritis and other inflammatory conditions, such as allergies.

Since grapeseed extract bolsters vitamin C, it is also important for strong bones. Although we don't think of vitamin C as a bone builder, it is actually essential for the formation of collagen, a component of bone. Collagen also provides the scaffolding beneath the skin; the loss of collagen can cause wrinkling. At least indirectly, grapeseed extract can help keep us stronger and looking younger through its effect on vitamin C.

POSSIBLE BENEFITS
- Antioxidant.
- Protects against atherosclerosis (hardening of the arteries).
- Anti-inflammatory.
- Cancer fighter.
- Helps build collagen.

HOW TO USE IT
Take up to two 100 mg. tablets twice daily. (I use a combination grapeseed extract/green tea extract product.)

GREEN TEA

• *Camellia sinensis* •

FACTS

Tea is the second most commonly consumed beverage in the world (water is first). Green tea, which is the beverage of choice in Japan, is a more lightly processed version of the black tea favored in the west, or the oolong tea popular in China. All forms of tea contain antioxidant flavonoids known as *polyphenols,* but the antioxidant activity of polyphenols in green tea are believed to be stronger. Antioxidants are important because they protect against *free radicals,* naturally occurring compounds in the body which, if not tightly controlled, can promote many different diseases including heart disease and cancer, as well as premature aging. Numerous animal studies have shown that various extracts from green tea can inhibit the initiation and progression of several different types of cancer. Researchers at Purdue University recently discovered that an antioxidant in green tea called *epigallocatechin gallate* can shut down an enzyme that cancer cells need to grow and divide. These findings are particularly important in light of the fact that several population studies have linked green-tea consumption with significantly lower rates of cancer. For example, even though Japanese men are heavier smokers than American men, they have a lower risk of lung cancer. Japanese researchers found that green-tea consumption cut lung cancer rates in mice exposed to a potent tobacco carcinogen. Other population studies have found that green tea appears to offer protection against cancer of the colon, esophagus, pancreas, stomach, and breast. Granted, there are no double-blind placebo controlled studies that definitively prove that green tea reduces cancer risk, but studies such as the ones I have cited are persuasive enough for me.

In addition, the polyphenols in green tea may protect against heart disease by preventing the oxidation of LDL. High blood levels of oxidized LDL cholesterol are linked to an increased risk of heart disease.

Tea contains about half the caffeine of coffee, so, if you are caffeine sensitive, don't drink it too close to bedtime.

POSSIBLE BENEFITS
- Keeps free radicals under control.
- Reduces risk of cancer.
- Helps prevent heart disease.

HOW TO USE IT

It's as simple as boiling water! Steep one tea bag in hot water for two minutes.

Green tea extract is available in tablets or capsules. For convenience's sake, I recommend a combination green tea/grapeseed extract tablet. Take 2 tablets daily. (One tablet is equal to $1^1/_2$ cups tea.)

GUARANA
• *Paulina cupana* •

FACTS

Recently, I had lunch with my friend Bill, who proudly announced that he had finally kicked the coffee habit. For as long as I had known him, Bill drank ten cups of strong, black coffee daily. Bill always seemed a bit jumpy and jittery, which I attributed to chronic caffeine overdose. I knew that Bill couldn't get through a day without coffee and, when he tried to go cold turkey, he always got a splitting headache. I asked him how he was finally able to give it up.

"I found this new supplement," he told me. "I don't need coffee anymore." The "new" supplement Bill had discovered was actually a well-known South American herb called *guarana*. In fact, it is one of the most popular herbs in the Southern Hemisphere. And guess what? Its primary ingredient is caffeine!

In South America, guarana is touted as a general tonic or revitalizer. It is widely used in soft drinks, cereals, and candy. Standardized guarana capsules are now available in the United States. Guarana has recently become popular in the United States among athletes and body builders looking for an extra boost. Each 500 mg. guarana capsule contains about one quarter the caffeine you would get in a cup of coffee.

Although caffeine does enhance physical performance and mental stamina, the problem is that caffeine highs can shortly give way to caffeine lows. Therefore, I do not believe in relying on caffeine as an energy source. Proponents of guarana contend that it contains other compounds that can help release the caffeine slowly, helping to maintain a more sustained effect. To me, caffeine in any form is a drug to be used with caution. Certainly, I am not against a cup or two of coffee in the morning, but overreliance on caffeine is not a good idea. The best way to reenergize the body is by eating well, taking the right supplements, and getting enough sleep.

POSSIBLE BENEFITS
- Provides energy boost.
- Improves concentration.
- Reputed to help athletes better recover from workouts.

HOW TO USE IT
Take one 500 mg. at breakfast and lunch. Do not use late in the day, since caffeine can interfere with sleep.

CAUTION: Caffeine constricts blood vessels, which is why it should not be used by people with heart disease, nor should it be taken by pregnant women.

GUGGULIPID
• *Cammiphora mukuk* •

FACTS

A gum extracted from the gaggle tree, which is native to India, has been a mainstay of Ayurvedic medicine for several centuries. Known as *guggulipid,* this natural plant extract has become a popular lipid-lowering agent in the United States. Several clinical studies show that guggulipid can significantly cut total cholesterol (about 25 percent) over a three-month period, as well as reduce high levels of triglycerides. High levels of cholesterol (over 200 mg./dl.), and triglycerides (over 200 mg./dl. in women and 400 mg./dl. in men) increase the risk of heart attack and stroke. Even better, guggulipid can boost the levels of good HDL cholesterol, which protects against heart disease, while cutting the amount of bad LDL cholesterol, which promotes heart disease.

Guggulipid is available as a single supplement and is often included in herbal formulas designed to promote cardiac health. One of the active ingredients in guggulipid is *guggulsterone,* a steroidlike compound, which is also sold separately.

POSSIBLE BENEFITS

- Helps correct poor blood lipids, which can cause heart disease.
- Raises HDL, which protects against heart disease.

HOW TO USE IT

Take one 500 mg. standardized guggulipid capsule with meals (standardized to 25 mg. guggulsterone) up to three times a day. I take a combination tablet of red yeast rice extract, guggulipid, and inositol hexanicotinate twice daily to keep my cholesterol in check.

HAWTHORNE
• *Crataegus oxyacantha* •

FACTS

Hawthorne berries have long been used to treat digestive problems and insomnia. In the late nineteenth century European physicians discovered that the berries from the hawthorne tree were also a cardiotonic. Today, standardized hawthorne extract is an approved treatment for heart disease in western Europe. Hawthorne is rich in *bioflavonoids,* compounds that are essential for vitamin C function and that also help strengthen blood vessels. This herb benefits the heart in many ways. It works as a *vasodilator,* that is, it increases the flow of blood and oxygen to the heart. It also lowers blood pressure, thus reducing the work required by the heart to pump blood through the body. At the same time, it helps strengthen the heart muscle. It also works as a diuretic, helping to rid the body of excess salt and water. Several German studies confirm that hawthorne can reduce symptoms of heart disease, boost energy levels, and help treat shortness of breath in patients suffering from heart failure and cardiac insufficiency. In other words, hawthorne can strengthen an ailing heart. It is also prescribed for patients who don't yet need digitalis, yet show signs of an *aging heart,* that is, a heart that does not pump as effectively as it once did. In several studies, heart patients taking hawthorne showed an increase in stamina and endurance when exercising. Researchers also noted an improvement in mood and sleeping patterns. Hawthorne has also been used successfully to treat angina or chest pain. As good as hawthorne may be, if you have a heart condition, you should be under the supervision of a physician who is knowledgeable in natural remedies. Do not discontinue your prescription medicine on your own to try an herbal supplement, or to add one to your drug regimen. In fact, if you are taking other heart drugs, if you take hawthorne, doses of other cardiac drugs may need to be adjusted.

What about people who want to prevent heart disease—is hawthorne for them? Many herbalists prescribe hawthorne as a cardiotonic to keep healthy hearts healthy. Although hawthorne is sold over the counter and there is absolutely no evidence that it is unsafe, I still think it makes sense to use this herb under the direction of a natural healer. There is a risk, albeit a small one, that people with an undiagnosed heart problem could exacerbate their problem by taking the wrong dose. Therefore, it is wise to err on the side of caution.

POSSIBLE BENEFITS
- Enhances cardiovascular health.
- Improves circulation.
- Can treat heart failure and angina.

HOW TO USE IT
Take up to three 200 mg. capsules daily with meals.

> **CAUTION:** Although most hawthorne preparations are safe, this herb is also available in a highly concentrated form that should be used only under medical supervision.

Personal Advice

I take a heart-health combination capsule of hawthorne and garlic extract, mixed tocopherol, cayenne, and Co Q10 twice daily. The capsule contains a touch of parsley seed oil to eliminate the garlic odor.

HORSE CHESTNUT

• *Aesculus hippocastum* •

FACTS

Although traditionally used as a remedy to bring down a fever and relieve cold symptoms, horse chestnut is being rediscovered in Europe for its ability to reduce swelling of varicose veins and soothe hemorrhoids. In Germany, an extract from the seed has been approved for poor circulation to the legs, leg cramps, swelling, and general "heaviness." A recent review article in the *Archives of Dermatology* (1998) analyzed 13 clinical studies involving the use of horse chestnut for *chronic venous insufficiency,* a condition characterized by swelling in the legs, or an aching, tired feeling in the legs when standing or walking. Most of the studies showed that horse chestnut helped to relieve symptoms better than a placebo, and even as well as a prescription drug made from a mixture of flavonoids. It takes about three weeks on average to experience positive results.

Horse-chestnut-seed extract has also been used as a sunscreen. According to folklore, carrying around the fruit of this tree in your pocket can prevent and cure arthritis. Many herbalists predict that, as the baby boomers approach middle age, horse chestnut will soon enjoy new popularity in the United States.

POSSIBLE BENEFITS
- A *vagotonic,* it strengthens and tones veins.
- Soothes irritated varicose veins.
- Promotes sweating and can help break a fever.

HOW TO USE IT

Take 10 to 15 drops extract daily, or one tablet as directed on package. (Look for products standardized to 50 mg. aescin, the active ingredient.)

Commercial preparations for external use are widely available. Use as directed on package. Apply gently.

CAUTION: Whole horse-chestnut seeds can be toxic, so do not attempt to make your own preparations.

The Great Garlic Mystery

During the Great Plague, some herbalists avoided this deadly disease by eating large amounts of garlic and wearing garlic strands around their necks. To this day, we don't know whether garlic's antibiotic properties protected these people against plague, or whether the foul stench of the herb discouraged others from getting close enough to spread their infection.

KAVA KAVA

• *Piper methysticum* •

FACTS

Touted as nature's valium, kava kava (or just kava) has become one of the most popular herbs in the United States. It has been used by the oceanic people of the South Pacific for thousands of years. Herbalists here have traditionally used it as a remedy for nervousness and insomnia. A natural muscle relaxant, it can also help relieve cramping due to muscle spasms. Kava was first discovered by explorer Captain James Cook, who gave this plant the botanical name "intoxicating pepper." The root of this plant is made into a popular beverage in Polynesia called *Sakau*. Offering guests a kava-laced beverage is considered the epitome of hospitality in the South Pacific. There's something to this ritual—kava immediately relaxes you without making you feel sluggish. I know from personal experience, as well as from numerous studies that, unlike standard tranquilizers, kava calms you down but usually does not affect mental alertness. Unlike alcohol, which can also have a calming effect, kava does not cause a hangover. Even though many people can take kava without feeling tired, some people may find that it makes them drowsy. Therefore, I recommend that it only be used at night when you are home for the evening. I could be accused of erring on the side of caution, but better to be safe than sorry.

POSSIBLE BENEFITS

- Helps you get a good night's sleep.
- Promotes relaxation.
- Helps reduce water retention.

HOW TO USE IT

Take 1 to 3 capsules daily as directed on package.
Take 10 to 20 drops of extract in juice or water daily.

CAUTION: Use only occasionally to relieve periods of stress or sleeplessness, up to two to three weeks at a time. Although rare, long-term use may cause liver damage and skin rashes. Do not exceed recommended dose or you may feel woozy. I do not recommend using kava with other prescription tranquilizers or anti-anxiety drugs unless under the direction of your physician or natural healer.

KUDZU

• *Pueraria thunbergiana* •

Ubiquitous throughout Asia and the southeastern United States, kudzu has been used in traditional Chinese medicine for thousands of years. In the United States, kudzu is being studied as a possible treatment for alcohol dependency. According to research conducted at Harvard Medical School, kudzu extract (containing two phytochemicals, *daidzein* and *daidzin*) can reduce alcohol addiction in hamsters specifically bred to develop a form of alcoholism similar to that found in humans. Both daidzein and daidzin are also found in soybeans, and are believed to have anticancer properties.

There are several kudzu products on the market that claim to help relieve the nasty symptoms of an alcohol-induced hangover. There are few scientific studies to suggest that kudzu is a cure for hangovers, but you can try it and see if it works for you. My best advice, however, is don't drink yourself sick. Stop after one or two drinks. If you have an alcohol-dependency problem, talk to a knowledgeable physician or healer about incorporating kudzu into your treatment.

POSSIBLE BENEFITS
- May reduce need for alcohol.
- May reduce nausea, headache and other symptoms typical of a hangover.

HOW TO USE IT
Take up to four 400 mg. capsules before or immediately following consumption of alcohol.

CAUTION: Although some herbalists believe that kudzu can lower blood-alcohol levels, this does not mean that as long as you take kudzu, you can drink without suffering the consequences. In particular, do not drink and drive under any circumstances.

LAVENDER

• *Lavendula augustifolia* •

FACTS

In the first edition of the *Herb Bible,* lavender was included in the list of Traditional Favorites, herbs that, because of their long history, are worthy of notice but could hardly be called hot. But, today, we know that lavender is much more than a pleasant fragrance to be used in sachets and potpourri—lavender can be powerful medicine. It has now earned a place on the Hot Hundred.

During the past decade, there has been a growing interest in *aromatherapy,* the use of scented essential oils to treat a wide array of ailments. Aromatherapy utilizes the power of scent to soothe, relax, and heal. Essential oils can be massaged into the skin, used in bath water or heated in a special lamp called an *aroma defuser.* Different scents evoke different emotions. Some are stimulants, others relieve stress or promote sleep. Some essential oils even have antiseptic properties, and were used to sterilize sick rooms in the days before antibiotics.

Recently, scientists have discovered that lavender oil has a soothing effect on the psyche. Researchers in England tested lavender oil on nursing-home patients suffering from insomnia, who normally use sleep medication. In a small six-week study, patients were first weaned from their medication for two weeks. For the next two weeks, they were not given any sleep aid. For the last two weeks, their rooms were perfumed with lavender oil. Although the patients had a great deal of difficulty sleeping during the second two weeks (after their medication had been discontinued), they had no trouble sleeping during the last two weeks. In fact, they slept as well with the lavender oil as they did on sleeping pills!

In Japan, scientists have discovered that inhaling lavender-oil vapor can prevent convulsions in mice. The scientists suspect that lavender may enhance the production of natural sedatives in the brains of mice as well as in those of humans.

POSSIBLE BENEFITS
- Induces calm.
- Promotes sleep.

HOW TO USE IT

Mix five drops of lavender oil in warm water for a
soothing bath. Put a few drops of oil in an aroma defuser.

Boil a quart of water, add a few drops, and inhale the
steam.

Apply a few drops of diluted oil to your skin. Buy an oil
preparation that is specially designed for use on skin.

LICORICE

• *Glycyrrhiza globra* •

FACTS

Licorice-flavored candy has been a popular confection for centuries.
The root of this plant, however, is also highly regarded for its medicinal
properties. The *Shennong Herbal,* a list of more than 365 plant drugs
compiled in China about two thousand years ago, lists licorice as a "superior" drug, meaning that it can be used over a long period of time
with no toxic effects. Culpeper wrote that this herb is "a fine medicine
for hoarseness."

More recently, foreign studies show that *glycyrrhizin,* the main active ingredient in licorice root, has anti-inflammatory, antiviral, and
anti-allergic properties. Licorice root is soothing for peptic ulcers, bladder ailments, and kidney ailments. It is also a good expectorant.
Licorice is a time-honored remedy for arthritis due to its anti-
inflammatory properties: It stimulates the production of two steroids,
cortisone and *aldosterone,* which help reduce inflammation. The Japanese are investigating glycyrrhizin as a possible cancer treatment. In the
United States, the National Cancer Institute is investigating *triter-*

penoids, compounds found in licorice root, for their ability to inhibit the growth of cancerous cells.

In Japan and China, glycyrrhizin has been used successfully to treat hepatitis B, a disease characterized by inflammation of the liver.

Licorice contains plant estrogens which, at high doses, bind to estrogen receptor sites on cells, thereby reducing the body's need for real estrogen. Herbalists include licorice in formulas to treat menopausal symptoms and menstrual disorders.

Licorice or, rather, glycrrihizin, can raise blood pressure in susceptible people. A new form of licorice minus glycyrrihizin, called *DGL,* has been used quite effectively to treat ulcers without producing the unwanted side effect of high blood pressure. It is an excellent substitute for over-the-counter antacids for either ulcer pain or heartburn. Since DGL does not contain glycyrrhizin acid, it is unlikely that it offers the full benefits of preparations containing the whole licorice root.

POSSIBLE BENEFITS
- Reduces pain of ulcers.
- Can relieve menopausal symptoms.
- Helps break up congestion due to colds.
- Soothes sore, hoarse throat.
- Reduces pain and stiffness from arthritis.
- May help retard growth of certain cancerous tumors.
- Used to treat hepatitis B.

HOW TO USE IT
Take up to 3 capsules daily.

CAUTION: Do not use licorice if you have *untreated* high blood pressure. The increased production of aldosterone can result in a rise in blood pressure. In large quantities, licorice can sap potassium from the body, which is extremely dangerous. Licorice candy does not offer the same benefits as preparations made from the root, but can cause an increase in blood pressure. Avoid use during pregnancy.

Personal Advice

Women who suffer from premenstrual syndrome should not use licorice during PMS, due to its ability to cause water retention or bloating.

MAITAKE MUSHROOM
• *Grifola frondosa* •

FACTS

This Japanese mushroom was so highly prized in ancient Japan that, in feudal times, it was exchanged for its weight in silver. Maitake contains *Beta-1,6 glucan,* a potent immune stimulant. Maitake stimulates the production of *T cells,* which defend the body against viruses and cancer. Japanese studies show that maitake extract can inhibit the growth of breast tumors and skin cancers in mice. In Japan and the United States, maitake is used along with other therapies to treat cancer and infectious diseases such as HIV. Interestingly, using maitake along with chemotherapy not only enhanced the effectiveness of the treatment, but resulted in fewer side effects, such as nausea and hair loss.

A small study conducted in New York showed that maitake supplements can produce a modest decline in high blood pressure. Japanese researchers say it also reduces high cholesterol and triglyceride levels, thereby protecting against heart disease and stroke. Animal studies suggest that maitake can reduce blood-glucose levels in diabetics, which may help prevent the devastating long-term consequences of diabetes, including blindness and nerve damage. Maitake is known as the *dancing mushroom,* because it grows in clusters that conjure the image of butterflies fluttering their wings.

POSSIBLE BENEFITS
- Stimulates immune function.
- Inhibits growth of cancerous tumors.
- Protects against heart disease and diabetes.

HOW TO USE IT

For general immune support, take 100 mg. standardized extract daily. If you already have cancer or a pre-existing problem, work with a physician.

MARIGOLD

• *Calendula officinalis* •

FACTS

Marigolds are not only beautiful flowers, but are also an important part of the herbal pharmacy. Traditional herbalists crush marigold petals in oil and apply it to cuts, burns, and other abrasions. For us modern day herbalists who prefer to buy our wares in natural food stores, there are wonderful marigold-based skin-care products sold under the botanical name calendula that can soothe and heal mild skin problems. Calendula is also used in herbal cleansers.

Marigold is an excellent source of *lutein,* a member of the carotenoid family that has been the subject of several groundbreaking scientific studies. Lutein is one of two carotenoids (*zeaxanthin* is the other) concentrated in the macular region of the eye. The *macula* is a small dimple that is responsible for central vision, required for focused activities like writing, sewing, driving, and for distinguishing color. Macular degeneration, the slow destruction of the macula, is the leading cause of blindness in people over forty. There is no cure or effective treatment for macular degeneration, but there is some evidence that lutein may help prevent it. In a study conducted at Harvard University, people who ate a diet rich in two dark green leafy vegetables, spinach and collard greens, had a substantially lower risk of developing age related macular degeneration. Since spinach and collard greens are excellent sources of both lutein and zeaxanthin, researchers concluded that these carotenoids may protect against macular degeneration.

Several lutein-based herbal supplements derived from marigold are being touted as vision protectors. Since macular degeneration can take years to develop, only time will tell if these products will be effective. However, there is no reason to believe that they won't.

POSSIBLE BENEFITS
- Used externally, soothes skin irritations, promotes healing.
- Taken orally, may help prevent macular degeneration.

HOW TO USE IT

Externally, apply calendula skin products directly to affected area.

Orally, take 6 to 20 mg. lutein daily, in capsules.

Personal Advice

People with light eyes are especially vulnerable to macular degeneration, which can be accelerated by exposure to sunlight. Be sure to wear sunglasses that block both UVA and UVB rays.

Garlic Gala

Since 1979, Gilroy, California, known as the "Garlic Capital of the World," has hosted the Annual Garlic Festival in celebration of the annual harvest. The event, which is held the last weekend in July, is a three-day food and wine tasting party drawing more than 140,000 garlic fans. Ninety percent of the U.S. garlic crop is grown in Gilroy and its environs. American humorist Will Rogers once described Gilroy as "the only town in America where you can marinate a steak by hanging it on the clothesline."

MARSHMALLOW

• *Althea officinalis* •

FACTS

King Charlemagne insisted that this herb be planted throughout his kingdom to ensure an abundant supply. Perhaps he had ulcers or colitis, because marshmallow is an old-time remedy for gastrointestinal disorders. It is high in mucilage, a substance that, when combined with water, develops a gel-like consistency. Mucilage can be very soothing to irritated mucous membranes. In fact, about eight hundred years after Charlemagne's death, Culpeper wrote that his son suffered from a disease called the "bloody flux," which the College of Physicians then called the *plague in the guts*. Culpeper treated his son by giving him "mallow bruised and boiled both in milk and drink." Two days later, his son was cured. Today, herbalists still use marshmallow to treat ulcers and colitis. It is also highly recommended for the raw, irritated feeling in the throat and chest often caused by bad coughs and bronchitis.

POSSIBLE BENEFITS

- Relieves pain caused by ulcers, enteritis, and colitis.
- Has a calming effect on the body.
- Can be a good expectorant for treating coughs.
- Soothes throat and chest irritation due to coughs and colds.

HOW TO USE IT

Take up to 3 capsules daily to relieve symptoms.

Mix 1 tablespoon of dried herb in 8 ounces boiling water. Strain. Drink up to 3 cups daily to relieve symptoms.

MILK THISTLE

• *Silybum marianum* •

FACTS

Milk thistle is extremely popular in Europe as a tonic for the liver, the body's second largest organ. Often referred to as the body's "chemical factory," the liver plays a critical role in maintaining good health. It produces bile, which is necessary for the breakdown of fats. It detoxifies poisons that enter our bloodstream, such as nicotine, alcohol, and pollutants such as carbon monoxide by breaking them down from potentially lethal substances into those that are less destructive to our bodies. The liver is also the site where vitamins A, D, E, and K are stored.

Milk thistle contains a flavonoid called *silymarin,* which has been shown to have a direct effect on liver cells. Also known as *vitamin P, flavonoids* are substances found in plants that often work in conjunction with vitamin C, and offer many other health benefits. Numerous European studies show that milk thistle enhances overall liver function, as well as stimulating the production of new liver cells. It also boosts the levels of *glutathione,* the powerful antioxidant that is found in highest concentration in the liver. Milk thistle has been used as an effective treatment for amanita mushroom poisoning, which kills its victim by destroying the liver. Treatment for mushroom poisoning will only work if it is given shortly after ingestion of the poisonous mushrooms. Silymarin has also been used to treat liver diseases, such as cirrhosis and hepatitis.

POSSIBLE BENEFITS
- Rejuvenates the liver.
- Increases production of bile used for breakdown of fats.
- Can protect against mushroom poisoning.

HOW TO USE IT

> Take one 140 mg. capsule up to three times daily. (Look for 70 percent silymarin.)

Personal Advice

This herb can be beneficial for those suffering from hepatitis or inflammation of the liver. It is also useful for people who have developed cirrhosis of the liver, a condition often caused by excessive alcohol intake. I also recommend it for anyone who smokes or is exposed to pollutants in the workplace. In addition, milk thistle is useful for people with signs of poor liver function, such as those with psoriasis and chronic yeast infection. I take a complete multivitamin and mineral with milk thistle for overall health.

MUIRA PUAMA
• *Ptychopetalum olacoides* •

FACTS

Also known as *potency wood*, this herb has recently gained popularity—and a bit of notoriety—as the hot new aphrodisiac from Brazil. It is reputed to stimulate libido and enhance sexual function. Although there are no scientific studies to back up these claims, there is a wealth of folklore, and a lot of hype, surrounding this herb. It is also used as a treatment for exhaustion.

POSSIBLE BENEFITS

> • Boosts sexual desire and function.

HOW TO USE IT

> Drink 1 cup tea daily.
> Take 1 to 3 capsules as directed on package.

NEEM

• *Azadirachta indica* •

FACTS

Neem is to Ayurvedic medicine what aspirin is to western medicine. It is a wonder drug that can be used to treat many common problems, from fever to headaches to skin disorders to fungal infections. No wonder it is known in Sanskrit as "the curer of all ailments." For 4,500 years, various parts of the neem tree have been a staple of the Ayurvedic pharmacy. Neem skin preparations are used to treat psoriasis, ringworm, athlete's foot, and warts. Today, neem is a common ingredient in numerous skin and hair products. For centuries, the bough of the neem plant was used in India as a toothbrush. Neem's natural antiseptic and anti-inflammatory compounds make it an excellent toothpaste and mouthwash; it is included in several commercial dental-care products.

Used orally, neem is a natural anti-inflammatory that can lower a fever, cure a headache, and reduce the pain of an earache. Neem also has antiviral properties, and has been used as a treatment for smallpox.

Neem is also used as a natural insecticide. Look for neem products at garden and lawn stores.

POSSIBLE BENEFITS
- Can soothe and heal skin disorders.
- Helps protect against gum disease.
- Natural anti-inflammatory.

HOW TO USE IT
Most neem products sold in the west are for external application. Apply neem skin lotion to affected areas up to three times daily. Use dental products as directed.

STINGING NETTLE

• *Urtica dioica* •

FACTS

Historically, this herb has been used to treat allergic symptoms and external wounds, such as bug bites. Today, this herb is gaining newfound popularity as a treatment for BPH (benign prostatic hypertrophy) in combination with such herbs as pygeum and saw palmetto. Nettle extract can inhibit the production of enzymes that contribute to the enlargement of the prostate. A natural diuretic, nettle is also useful for problems of the urinary tract and kidney stones.

POSSIBLE BENEFITS

- Alleviates stuffy nose, watery eyes, and other symptoms of hay fever.
- Helps relieve symptoms of enlarged prostate.

HOW TO USE IT

Take up to 3 capsules daily (up to 300 mg. per day). For hay fever, it is best to take the capsules in smaller doses throughout the day.

Mix 5 to 10 drops extract in liquid daily.

CAUTION: Do not eat uncooked plants—they can cause kidney damage and symptoms of poisoning. Handle plants with care. The bristly hairs act like tiny hypodermic needles, injecting an irritant under the skin. Avoid this herb if you have diabetes, kidney problems, or heart disease. I take a combination capsule of saw palmetto, pygeum, and nettle extract, plus zinc and beta sistosterols and soy isoflavone complex for my prostate health twice daily. I recommend it to all men over forty.

Personal Advice

I take tablets containing stinging nettles, pygium, saw palmetto, zinc, selenium, and beta sisterol (from soy).

OAT FIBER

• *Avena sativa* •

FACTS

Long before breakfast meant a bowl of sugar-coated, artificially flavored cereal, our "less-enlightened" ancestors thrived on whole grains. The grain from the oat plant is not only nutritious, but serves another important purpose: It is one of the most effective ways to reduce serum cholesterol. Rich in a gum called *beta glucan,* 2 to 3 ounces of oat fiber per day in a low-fat diet can reduce cholesterol by 5 to 10 percent. Oat extract is a natural relaxant, and is also excellent for indigestion. No part of the oat plant need go to waste: The dried coarse stem or straw can be used in baths to soothe hemorrhoids and to revitalize sore, aching feet.

POSSIBLE BENEFITS
- Good for gas and upset stomach.
- Helps prevent heart disease by reducing cholesterol.
- Good source of vitamin B.
- Good for skin and hemorrhoids.
- Extract has a calming effect on the body.

HOW TO USE IT
Eat foods rich in oat fiber.
For indigestion, take 10 to 20 drops extract up to 3 times daily to relieve symptoms. The straw is used in external preparations in baths, sitz baths for hemorrhoids, and foot baths.

Personal Advice

Gradually increase the amount of oat bran you eat every day, giving your body time to adjust to the change in diet. If you take in too much at once, you may suffer from cramps and gas. Drinking 6 to 8 glasses of filtered water daily will help eliminate this problem.

OLIVE LEAF EXTRACT
• *Olea europaea* •

F A C T S

The olive branch may be a universal sign of peace, but the extract from the olive leaf is a potent fighter against disease. Olive leaf contains a compound called *oleuropein acid,* a natural microbe buster, which is effective against numerous viruses, bacteria, and fungi. Physicians report success in treating a wide variety of ailments with olive leaf extract. According to James R. Privatera, M.D., who routinely uses olive leaf extract in his practice, this natural remedy is particularly good for people with hard-to-treat viral infections, such as Epstein-Barr disease, chronic fatigue syndrome, and herpes. It has even helped relieve symptoms of people with AIDS. Notably, it helps bolster the immune system, giving the body more ammunition to fight infection. Olive leaf extract is not a cure-all, but it can help reduce debilitating fatigue, pain, and other symptoms that can interfere with the quality of life. Olive leaf extract helps destroy viruses in two important ways. First, it interferes with the ability of the virus to replicate, which prevents the virus from spreading. Second, it stimulates the immune system to produce more disease-fighting cells. In particular, olive leaf extract seems to be good for patients who have suffered through chronic illness, and need an extra boost to regain their health. Along with a health-conscious lifestyle, olive leaf extract can help reduce viral load in the body as well as restore a flagging immune system.

Olive leaf extract is also an excellent treatment for old-fashioned colds and flus, which cannot be treated with antibiotics. The only recourse is to allow them to run their course, which may be a bit shorter if you use natural immune stimulants such as olive leaf extract, elderberry extract, and plenty of hot chicken soup.

Similar to olive oil, olive leaf extract is good for your heart. Animal studies show it can lower high blood pressure and reduce high levels of blood cholesterol.

POSSIBLE BENEFITS

- Protects against chronic viral infections.
- Treats yeast infections.

HOW TO USE IT

If you are currently sick with a cold, flu, or viral infection, take three 500 mg tablets every four hours. If your fever persists more than 24 hours, or if you suffer any untoward symptoms, don't self-medicate. Call your physician or natural healer immediately. If you are run down, or have been exposed to a cold or flu, fortify your immune system by taking one 500 mg. tablet daily.

ONION

• *Allium cepa* •

FACTS

The everyday onion is one of the oldest and most versatile of remedies. Long before commercial cold remedies, herbalists used a syrup made from the juice of an onion mixed with honey to alleviate congestion. Culpeper recommends it "to help an inveterate cough, and expectorate tough phlegm." I've tried it myself, and the stuff works as well as many over-the-counter cough medicines, without some of the unpleasant side effects, like drowsiness or nervousness. Onion is also excellent for the digestion.

An onion a day may also keep the cardiologist away. Studies show that people who eat a medium onion daily can lower their overall cholesterol and raise their HDL. Onion has also been shown to lower blood pressure and help prevent blood clots. A recent study by the National Cancer Institute showed that people who consume diets high in allium vegetables, such as onion, are diagnosed with stomach cancer less often than those who don't. Onion contains many cancer-fighting compounds, including quercetin which, in test tube studies, has inhibited the action of many different carcinogens. Onion is also rich in selenium, a mineral that has recently been shown to reduce the risk of prostate, lung, and breast cancer. Selenium is also believed to protect against stroke. In fact, the regions of the world with the lowest selenium content in the soil have the per capita highest rate of stroke.

A roasted onion can be used as a poultice for earaches. Onion is believed to be a natural source of energy, and some people swear that an onion per day can prevent hair loss. Applied directly to the skin, onion has special healing properties. Salted onions are useful for troublesome warts. Onion juice rubbed between the toes 2 to 3 times daily can cure athlete's foot. A mixture of 1 to 2 teaspoons onion juice with 1 teaspoon vinegar can fade unsightly liver spots or dark blemishes.

POSSIBLE BENEFITS

- Protects against cancer.
- Good expectorant.
- Relieves symptoms of common cold.
- Good for digestion.
- Helps prevent heart disease and cancer.
- Antifungal—good for warts.
- Good antiseptic.

HOW TO USE IT

Take 1 teaspoon of juice 3 to 4 times daily. To make onion juice, puree one raw onion in a blender or food processor and strain through cheesecloth. Store in the refrigerator.

For colds, mix warm juice with 2 teaspoons honey.

Rub juice on warts or between toes to fight athlete's foot. Can be used as antiseptic on skin wounds.

CAUTION: If you're breast-feeding an infant, stay clear of onions, because they could cause the baby to suffer from colic.

Try eating a parsley sprig to avoid onion breath. Chlorophyll tablets also can help eliminate odor. According to folklore, onion helps restore sexual potency!

OREGANO

• *Oreganum vulgare* •

FACTS

Often confused with the milder, sweeter marjoram, true oregano is a leafy perennial of the mint family native to the Mediterranean. The ancient Greeks and Romans valued oregano both to flavor food and to act as a medicine. It is believed that oregano was used for medicine as far back as the time of the cave man! Ancient Greeks used crushed oregano leaves on wounds and sore joints. Greek healers prescribed it for parasites and other infections. The Romans popularized oregano throughout Europe where oregano oil was used to disinfect a sick room. Even though they were unaware of the existence of germs, they did know that disease was often spread through physical contact with the sick.

Recently, modern herbalists have rediscovered oil of oregano as a treatment for fungal infections, warts, psoriasis, and even the common cold. Oregano oil contains two natural antiseptic compounds, *carvacol* and *thymol*. It is also a natural anti-inflammatory, which can help promote healing of skin wounds and muscle strains.

POSSIBLE BENEFITS
- Natural disinfectant and antimicrobial.
- May help you beat a cold or flu.
- May promote healing of skin wounds.

HOW TO USE IT
For an active infection, take up to six oregano-oil capsules daily for up to two weeks.

Mix 5 to 10 oregano drops in liquid. Drink up to 2 cups
daily.
Place a few drops of oil directly on warts or skin
wounds. Use daily until healed.

Personal Advice

Buy only products that are true oregano (*oregano vulgare*). The spice
you buy in the supermarket that is sold as oregano is often a form of
marjoram and, although it's great in tomato sauce or on pizza, it does
not have the potency of real oregano.

Osha

• *Ligusticum porteri* •

FACTS

This herb was originally used by western Native Americans to treat
colds, flu, and upper respiratory infections. Osha is purported to be an
immune builder, that is, it helps the body ward off viral infections.
Look for osha in immune-boosting formulas that also include echinacea, astragalus, and lomatuum root.

POSSIBLE BENEFITS
• May enhance immune function.

HOW TO USE IT
Take 1 capsule up to 3 times daily. Mix 20 to 30 drops
extract in liquid up to 3 times daily.

PAPAYA
....
• *Carica papaya* •

FACTS

If you can't get through a day without popping an antacid, this is the herb for you. Papaya contains a substance called *papain,* which is chemically similar to *pepsin,* an enzyme that helps digest protein in the body. It is a safe and natural digestive aid. I know that it's easy enough to buy an over-the-counter alternative, but it is certainly not any better. In fact, in a lot ways, it is much worse. If you take too many antacids, you run the risk of the *rebound effect,* that is, your body will respond by producing even more acid, which will cause even more gastrointestinal problems. Papaya juice or tablets, however, can be taken freely without any fear of rebounding. The fruit is also delicious and very popular in Hawaii.

POSSIBLE BENEFITS
• Aids in the breakdown and metabolism of protein.
• Helps relieve indigestion.

HOW TO USE IT
Drink papaya juice, or chew 1 to 2 tablets daily after eating to relieve symptoms.

Personal Advice
Papaya is commercially available in a delicious, chewable tablet form. Dried papaya slices are also an excellent way to take advantage of this herb's benefits.

PARSLEY

• *Petroselinum sativum* •

FACTS

Every night after dinner, my grandmother used to make herself a cup of parsley tea. She'd take a few sprigs of parsley, steep them in hot water for several minutes, and then sip the tea slowly. When I asked her why she did it, she shrugged and said that her grandmother told her to. Her grandmother knew what she was doing. Parsley is a natural antispasmodic: in other words, it's great for the digestion. It relieves gas and is a natural diuretic. It is also a good expectorant and can be used for coughs and asthma.

Although parsley is often used as a garnish, don't leave it on the plate! Parsley is a member of the *umbelliferous* vegetable family, which contains powerful anticancer compounds.

Herbalists used parsley oil to regulate menstruation and induce abortion. Rubbed on the scalp, parsley oil purportedly stimulates hair growth.

POSSIBLE BENEFITS
- Helps settle the stomach after a meal.
- Helps clear congestion due to coughs and colds.
- Protects against cancer.

HOW TO USE IT
Eat raw, or steep chopped leaves and stems in hot water. Drink daily.

CAUTION: Pregnant women should not take parsley juice or oil.

Personal Advice

Parsley is a wonderful source of chlorophyll, nature's own breath freshener. Try it after eating onions or garlic.

PASSION FLOWER
• *Passiflora incarnata* •

FACTS

This herb is one of nature's best tranquilizers. It relieves muscle tension and other manifestations of extreme anxiety. It is especially good for nervous insomnia: the kind that keeps you lying in bed worrying until the wee hours of the morning. Since the tryptophan scare, in which a contaminated batch of this essential amino acid was linked to several deaths, passionflower has become very popular as a safe, natural alternative to help promote a good night's sleep. Herbalists often recommend passionflower for times of extreme emotional upset.

POSSIBLE BENEFITS
- Has a calming effect.
- Can relieve headaches due to nervous tension.
- Good for muscle spasms due to nerves.

HOW TO USE IT
Mix 15 to 60 drops of extract in liquid as needed daily.

CAUTION: This herb may cause sleepiness in some people, and should not be used before driving or operating machinery. Do not take during pregnancy.

Pau D'Arco

• *Tabecuia impetiginosa* •

FACTS

From Brazil comes the bark of this tree, which has numerous health benefits. It's an old-time remedy for candida, athlete's foot, and other annoying fungal infections. Research in South America and the United States shows that *lapachol,* an extract from the tree's bark, contains active ingredients found to be effective against some forms of cancer. However, lapachol is not considered a viable cancer treatment because tests on humans conducted by the National Cancer Institute indicated that high levels can cause many undesirable side effects. Another study done at the Naval School of Health Sciences in Bethesda, Maryland, in 1974 found that lapachol is quite useful against parasitic infection. Pau d'arco seems to lower blood-sugar levels, which may help prevent diabetes. On top of everything else, this herb is reputed to be good for the digestion!

POSSIBLE BENEFITS
- Helps cure fungal infections.
- Helps fight parasitic infection.
- Promotes good digestion.
- Lowers blood sugar.

HOW TO USE IT
Take up to 3 capsules daily.
Mix 25 to 40 drops extract in liquid up to 3 times daily.
Drink 1 cup tea up to 3 times daily.

PEPPERMINT
• *Mentha piperita* •

FACTS

Peppermint is one of the oldest and best-tasting home remedies for indigestion. Studies show that peppermint lessens the amount of time food spends in the stomach by stimulating the gastric lining. It also relaxes the stomach muscles and promotes burping. Peppermint is excellent for heartburn and stomachache, as well as nausea and vomiting. Migraine headaches, which are frequently accompanied by nausea, are often relieved by peppermint. This herb has a calming effect on the body and can help soothe a nagging cough.

POSSIBLE BENEFITS
- Antispasmodic—good for cramps and stomach pain.
- Relieves gas.
- Aids in digestion.
- Can help reduce sick feeling typical of migraine headaches.
- Can help with insomnia.

HOW TO USE IT
Drink 1 cup of tea daily. Many commercial teas are available.

Personal Advice

This is an excellent substitute for regular coffee and tea—and better tasting, too. For a headache, try a strong cup of peppermint tea and lie down for 15 to 20 minutes. I think that it works better than aspirin or acetaminophen. Considering all the things that peppermint can do, no home medicine cabinet should be without it! Peppermint extract has been used for centuries for colic in infants and for older children. Check with your pediatrician before giving this or any other herb to your child. Many restaurants give their patrons peppermint candy after a multicourse meal to aid digestion. That is why better hotels put peppermint candies on your pillow during turndown service. A good night's rest is guaranteed!

PINE-BARK EXTRACT
• *Pinus maritima* •

FACTS

Pine-bark extract is a rich source of *flavonoids,* a family of more than 4000 compounds found in plants, many of which are potent antioxidants. Traditional healers have used pine bark preparations to treat a wide range of ailments, from flu to circulatory disorders to inflammatory conditions, such as rheumatoid arthritis and colitis. Today, pine bark is being rediscovered by modern scientists who are reaffirming what traditional herbalists have known for centuries: pine bark is strong medicine.

The power of pine bark is due to its high flavonoid content. *Flavonoids* help to control nitric oxide, a chemical that regulates the muscular tone of blood vessels, which is key to circulation. If nitric-oxide levels get too high, blood flow could be interrupted to key organs, resulting in serious problems such as heart attack, stroke, and impotence.

Pine bark is a natural anti-inflammatory. Since inflammation is involved in so many different health problems related to aging—from gum disease to gastrointestinal problems to cancer—it is important to counteract the inflammatory process within the body by maintaining a high level of flavonoids through food and supplements.

In test-tube studies, pine bark has been shown to be a powerful immune enhancer. Researchers tested a patented form of pine-bark extract (called *Pycnogenol*) in a mouse model of an HIV-like virus and alcoholism, two conditions that can destroy a healthy immune system. In both experiments, pine-bark extract boosted immune function in the immune-compromised mice by increasing the production of *interluekin*-2, which promotes the activity of disease-fighting T-cells and lymphocytes. In healthy mice, pine-bark extract stimulated the production of cancer-fighting natural killer (NK) cells.

The flavonoids in pine bark enhance the action of vitamin C in the body. Therefore, every time you take pine-bark supplements, you are not only getting the benefit of flavonoids, but at the same time, are maximizing the positive effects of vitamin C.

Since pine bark improves blood flow everywhere in the body, including the brain, it can help improve concentration and enhance alertness. A recent study suggests that it may even improve athletic performance. Researchers at the California State University at Chico reported that pine-bark extract increases endurance time by 21 percent in both men and women during exercise.

POSSIBLE BENEFITS

- Protects against heart disease and stroke. Keeps immune system strong.
- May relieve inflammation from arthritis.

HOW TO USE IT

Take one 30 mg. capsule daily.

Personal Advice

Some people find pine bark to be a stimulant, so take it in the morning. You may find that pine bark will wake you up as well as your morning cup of coffee.

PSYLLIUM
• *Plantago psyllium* •

FACTS

A leading cereal manufacturer recently discovered what herbalists have known for decades: Ground seeds from the psyllium plant are one of the highest sources of dietary fiber to be found in any food. For centuries, psyllium has been used to treat ulcers, colitis, and constipation.

We now know that it helps clear the body of excess cholesterol: This herb is now touted as a preventive against heart disease. It may also raise the level of beneficial HDLs (good cholesterol) in the blood.

POSSIBLE BENEFITS

- An excellent laxative that offers relief from hemorrhoidal irritation.
- May help prevent heart disease.

HOW TO USE IT

Mix 1 teaspoon of ground seeds or powder in 1 cup liquid, and drink 2 to 3 times daily.

CAUTION: Psyllium can cause allergic reactions in sensitive individuals. If you are highly allergic to many other substances, I recommend that you avoid this one, or certainly check with your allergist before taking it. If you want to include psyllium in your diet, you should start slowly, allowing your body time to get used to the increased fiber. Be patient. In two to three weeks, it will. Too much at one time could cause gasiness and stomach discomfort. It is important to drink 8 to 10 glasses of water throughout the day when you are using this substance to increase its efficiency. If you develop any allergic symptoms, discontinue use. Do not use psyllium to treat an ulcer or colitis without checking with your physician.

Hamlet on Herbs

Rosemary is an ancient folk remedy for improving memory. In *Hamlet* Shakespeare wrote "That's Rosemary, that's for remembrance; I pray you, love, remember."

PYGEUM
....
• *Pygeum Africanum* •

FACTS

When I first wrote the *Herb Bible* ten years ago, the state of a man's prostate was not considered a topic suitable for polite discussion. What a difference ten years makes! As baby boomers enter their middle years, the same generation that has dealt frankly with formerly taboo topics, such as sex and menopause, are now dealing with prostate health with a new openness and honesty. In fact, I was at a dinner party recently when a man leaned across the table and said, not in a whisper, but quite audibly, "So, Earl, what should I be taking for my prostate!" And nobody seemed surprised.

The prostate is a small, walnut-shaped gland that surrounds the part of the urethra that is located under the bladder. At around age forty, hormonal changes cause the prostate to enlarge. Although it is usually not serious, benign prostate hypertrophy (BPH) can be extremely uncomfortable, causing an increased frequency of urination and the inability to empty the bladder completely, among other unpleasant symptoms.

For centuries, traditional healers in Africa have used the bark of the *pygeum tree,* an evergreen native to Africa, to treat prostate problems. In 1966, Dr. Jacques Debat acquired the first patent for a pygeum-bark extract and introduced the herb to Europe, where it is now used routinely to treat enlarged prostate, often along with other herbs, such as saw palmetto and nettle root.

Pygeum bark contains *phytosterols,* steroidlike compounds that are natural anti-inflammatories. It contains other chemicals that can help control the production of potent forms of testosterone, which not only cause enlargement of the prostate, but can increase the risk of prostate cancer, a condition unrelated to BPH.

Pygeum has become so popular that *Herbalgram,* a magazine that follows the herb industry, recently reported that pygeum bark is being overharvested, which could not only lead to a shortage of this valuable herb, but put the species at risk of extinction.

POSSIBLE BENEFITS
- Works well with other herbs to control BPH symptoms.

HOW TO USE IT
I recommend a combination formula containing pygeum, saw palmetto, nettles, beta sitosterol, zinc, lycopene, and soy isoflavones. Take 4 tablets daily.

RASPBERRY LEAVES
• *Rubus idaeus* •

FACTS

Back in the days when midwives were the primary healthcare providers to women, and natural childbirth was the only way to have a baby, the leaf of the raspberry bush was the herb of choice. Women routinely brewed it into a tea to drink during their last two months of pregnancy to tone their uterine muscles for labor and delivery. After birth, raspberry tea was taken for several weeks to help the uterus return to normal. It is also excellent for menstrual cramps. Warm raspberry-leaf tea is also soothing for throat irritations and canker sores, and is also effective against diarrhea.

POSSIBLE BENEFITS
- Prepares the uterus for childbirth, may help shorten labor.
- Good for sore throats and fever blisters.
- Alleviates menstrual cramps.

HOW TO USE IT

Mix 1 teaspoon dried herb in 1 cup warm water. Drink
daily.
Mix 15 to 30 drops extract up to 3 times daily. Drink
warm for best results.
Drink 1 cup tea daily.

CAUTION: Do not use until the last two months of pregnancy, and then only under the supervision of a qualified health practitioner.

RED CLOVER

• *Trifolium pratense* •

FACTS

Traditionally, the blossoms of this plant were used as a tonic taken in the spring to promote good health and peace of mind. It contains small amounts of silica, choline, calcium, and lecithin—all essential for normal body function. It works as a muscle relaxer and also is a good expectorant. It is an old-time remedy for eczema.

Combined with other herbs, red clover is used to prevent and treat cancer. Red clover is rich in phytoestrogens, weak estrogenlike compounds that can block the effect of more potent estrogens in the body by competing with them for receptor sites on cells. Since real estrogen can stimulate the growth of existing cancers that are estrogen sensitive—for example, breast cells—weaker plant estrogens can help prevent the spread of existing cancers by keeping real estrogen away from these sensitive cells. In the 1940s, this herb received a good deal of notoriety because it was included in herbal healer Harry Hoxsey's anticancer formula, dubbed the "red-clover combination." Hoxsey ran a chain of cancer clinics that were under frequent attack by the American Medical

Association. At that time, the only legitimate treatments for cancer were surgery or radiation. Although the medical establishment portrayed Hoxsey as a quack, we now know that many of the herbs included in his formula have antitumor properties. Modern research also validates the use of other herbs, such as Madagascar periwinkle for leukemia and Pacific hew for uterine and prostate cancer. Although Hoxsey's formula may not have been a cure-all for cancer, he was a pioneer in incorporating folklore treatments in modern-day cancer therapy.

Red clover is also being used as a treatment for the side effects of menopause. As estrogen levels dip in the body, weaker plant estrogens can relieve many of the symptoms caused by estrogen deficiency, such as hot flashes. *Isoflavones,* a type of phytoestrogen, have also been shown to have a bone-sparing effect, meaning they can help prevent osteoporosis by preventing the loss of calcium.

POSSIBLE BENEFITS
- Helps prevent cancer.
- Used to treat menopausal symptoms.
- Good for skin inflammations.
- Relaxes the body.

HOW TO USE IT
Take up to 3 capsules daily.
Mix 10 to 30 drops of extract in warm liquid daily.

CAUTION: Please seek professional help before using this or any other herb to treat tumors and cancer. Any cancer treatment should be done under the supervision of a physician.

RED YEAST RICE

• *Meniscus purpureus* •

FACTS

Red yeast rice, the "new" treatment for high cholesterol, is actually an ancient Chinese remedy that dates back to 800 C.E.! Chinese chefs use red yeast rice as a coloring agent to give Peking duck and roast pork their characteristic red color. It is also used to preserve food and ferment rice wine. Unlike many natural remedies that rely on anecdotal evidence, red yeast rice is backed by solid, scientific study. Several well-done, double-blind, placebo-controlled studies involving thousands of patients have shown that for people with high cholesterol (over 230 mg./dl.), red yeast rice is a highly effective cholesterol-lowering agent that can cut cholesterol by up to 15 percent. It not only reduces the bad LDL cholesterol, but also cuts triglyceride levels. However, red yeast rice worked best when combined with a low-fat diet and an exercise program. Marketed under the name *Cholestin,* red yeast rice has taken the United States by storm. However, even though it is sold over the counter, it is a potent drug, and is not safe for everyone. Although side effects are rare, there is a slight chance of negative side effects. In particular, red yeast rice should be avoided by people with liver problems, heavy drinkers (more than three drinks daily), pregnant women or nursing women, transplant patients, and seriously ill people (unless used under a doctor's supervision).

POSSIBLE BENEFITS
• By normalizing high blood lipids, may prevent heart attack and stroke.

HOW TO USE IT
Take two 600 mg. capsules twice daily.

Personal Advice

For many people, red yeast rice may work as well as prescription medicines but with far fewer side effects. For an added boost, combine it with other herbal cholesterol-lowering agents. I take a combination of red yeast rice extract, guggulipid, inositol hexanicotinate, B[8], folate, and soy isolates twice daily to normalize my cholesterol.

REISHI MUSHROOM

• *Ganoderma lucidum* •

FACTS

Reishi is so highly regarded in China that it has been dubbed "the medicine of kings." This delicious mushroom, which is popular in Asian cuisines, is well known for its heart-healthy properties. Reishi can lower high cholesterol and high blood pressure, two well-known risk factors for heart disease and stroke. Recently, reishi has been studied for its anti-cancer properties. It contains a compound called *Beta D glucan*, which can stimulate the production of cancer-fighting immune cells. Although there have been anecdotal reports of reishi extract used successfully to treat cancer, there have not been any clinical studies to date.

Other studies have confirmed that this mushroom has a strong antihistamine action, which can help control allergies. It is also a natural anti-inflammatory and muscle relaxant, good for treating the aches and pains associated with arthritis and muscle strains.

In Japan, reishi is a popular treatment for stress-related ailments. For centuries, Asian healers have prescribed it for anxiety and insomnia.

POSSIBLE BENEFITS
- May help enhance immune function.
- May be useful for arthritic pain.

HOW TO USE IT
Take 1 capsule up to 3 times daily.

ROSEMARY

• *Rosmarinus officinalis* •

FACTS

Whoever first coined the adage "Everything old is new again," must have had rosemary in mind. In the first edition of the *Herb Bible,* rosemary was included among traditional favorites. As with a handful of other "old-timers," rosemary has been elevated to the Hot Hundred, thanks to recent scientific discoveries.

For thousands of years, rosemary has been used in cooking, traditional medicine, and touted as a memory enhancer. In ancient Greece, students wore sprigs of rosemary in their hair because they believed it would sharpen their memory.

In modern times, rosemary has been used as a natural preservative that can keep fats from going rancid. Rosemary contains *carnosic acid,* an antioxidant that can protect against *oxidation,* the process by which food goes bad. Within our bodies, oxidation is a process that gives rise to *free radicals,* highly reactive substances that cause damage to healthy cells. Chronic damage inflicted by free radicals is a leading cause of cancer, heart disease, macular degeneration, and premature aging. Free radicals are also believed to be involved in the slow but steady destruction of brain tissue which gives rise to normal age-related memory problems (the "Where did I put the car keys?" variety), as well as the more serious Alzheimer's disease.

Rosemary's disease-fighting power was underscored by a study conducted at Penn State—appropriately called the Rosemary Study—which found that a diet supplemented with dried rosemary could protect rats that were fed a strong carcinogen from developing cancer. The rats were given a cancer-causing agent known to bind to breast cells, causing them to turn cancerous. The study showed that in rats fed rosemary, the carcinogen was much less likely to bind to breast cells than in rats that were not. Researchers speculate that rosemary may have a similar effect in humans.

There may also be a scientific explanation for rosemary's reputation as a brain booster. Rosemary contains chemicals called *acetyl-cholinestrase inhibitors,* which prevent the breakdown of a chemical produced by the brain, called *acetylcholine.* Acetylcholine deficiency has been implicated in Alzheimer's disease and other memory problems.

POSSIBLE BENEFITS
- Protects against free radical attack.
- May reduce the risk of breast cancer.
- May help preserve memory.

HOW TO USE IT

Take two 500 mg. standardized rosemary capsules daily.

Personal Advice

Use a sprig of fresh rosemary in your cooking!

SAINT JOHN'S WORT

• *Hypericum perforatum* •

FACTS

Since the publication of the first edition of the *Herb Bible,* St. John's wort (also known as *hypericum*) has emerged as *the* herb of choice for depression. In fact, it has been dubbed "nature's prozac," because of its success in treating mild to moderate depression. In Germany, St. John's wort is the number-one prescription drug for depression, and it is widely used throughout Europe. Through the years, this herb has also been used as a mild tranquilizer and as a treatment for insomnia. There have been numerous clinical studies conducted on St. John's wort in Europe. An article in the *British Medical Journal* reviewed twenty-three clinical trials of St. John's wort, and concluded that it worked as well as many prescription antidepressants, but with fewer of the unpleasant side effects, including dry mouth, constipation, and dizziness, at least at lower doses. In the United States, the National Institutes of Health are coordinating a multicenter study to investigate the use of St. John's wort as an antidepressant. As usual, the scientific establishment is well behind the curve—millions of people are already taking St. John's wort with good result. Although St. John's wort has been used in Europe for several decades, there have not been any official studies investigating long-term use of this herb. Since there have not been any problems reported as yet in Europe, it is reasonable to conclude that this herb is at least as safe as prescription antidepressants, if not safer.

St. John's wort is steeped in superstition and lore. If you rub the petals of this flower between your fingers, red resin will ooze out, leaving a stain on your hand. Perhaps that is why, according to a legend dating back to the Middle Ages, this plant sprang from John the Baptist's blood when he was beheaded. Early Christians believed that this herb could chase away evil spirits. Since depression and other mood disorders were often attributed to witchcraft and demonic possession, it is not surprising that herbalists believed that St. John's wort was an antidote to black magic.

St. John's wort is also a muscle relaxer, and has been used to treat menstrual cramps. It is a good expectorant as well. In Europe, it is also a popular remedy for gastrointestinal disorders, such as gastric ulcers. Externally, it is an antiseptic and a painkiller for burns and irritations. Ointments are also used for rheumatism and sciatica or back pain. Researchers at two of the world's leading medical institutions—New York University and the Weizman Institute of Science in Israel—found that two of its main constituents, hypericin and pseudohypericin, were found to inhibit the growth of retroviruses in animals, including HIV, the AIDS virus. Although the results of these studies are promising, a synthetic form of hypericin is just now being tested on HIV-infected patients. More studies are needed to determine if this herb can be useful against AIDS.

Recently, St. John's wort has been touted as an herb that promotes weight loss. Some researchers believe that, similar to Prozac, St. John's wort helps regulate serotonin levels in the brain, which can help to control appetite. There are no studies, however, to support this claim yet.

POSSIBLE BENEFITS

- Treatment for depression.
- Has a calming effect.
- Relieves uterine cramping.
- Promotes healing of skin wounds.
- Helps the body fight viral infection.

HOW TO USE IT

Take up to three 300 mg. capsules daily. (Look for .3% hypericin.)

Mix 10 to 15 drops of extract in liquid daily.

CAUTION: Do not take St. John's wort with other antidepressants unless you are under medical supervision.

Personal Advice

If you are severely depressed, are unable to function, or are suicidal, don't self-medicate. You must be treated by a knowledgeable physician or natural healer. Although St. John's wort works well for many people, it does not work for everyone. In some cases, other treatment, including prescription medication, may be required. Store your St. John's wort carefully. Keep it in a dark, cool place away from direct light and heat. I take a potent nutraceutical combination of St. John's wort and polyphenol extract. It works in just 2 to 3 days. Two tablets are taken daily for the first month, then one thereafter. I find it helps me cope with stress and is a wonderful muscle relaxant.

SARSAPARILLA
....
• *Smilax officinalis* •

FACTS

Since it was brought to Europe from the New World by Spanish traders in the 1600s, there has been a mystique surrounding this controversial herb. Originally, sarsaparilla was used to treat syphilis, but it soon became known as a tonic for male sexual potency. Some herbalists claim that its steroidlike compounds—*saponin glycosides*—actually contain male hormones. This has never been proven, although these substances appear to stimulate the body's metabolic processes. Because it promotes urination and sweating, sarsaparilla has been touted as a blood purifier by old-time herbalists who believed that toxins are released through bodily secretions. At the very least, these properties mean that the herb can be useful in cooling down the body or breaking a fever.

Recently, this herb has been marketed as a "male herb" that can increase muscle mass in much the same way that steroids do. There is no evidence to back up this claim. At the turn of the century, the claims for this herb were no less grandiose. In fact, it was sold as a cure-all for nearly every malady known to man—and woman, for that matter! Because of a lack of sound research, when it comes to sarsaparilla, it's difficult to separate fact from fiction. All we know is that for centuries, different cultures have utilized this herb often in surprisingly similar ways. For example, Europeans used sarsaparilla as an anti-inflammatory for rheumatoid arthritis, osteoarthritis, and also as a treatment for urinary tract disorders; so did the Chinese. Native Americans also used this herb for urinary problems, arthritis, and as a rejuvenating tonic. In fact, until 1950, sarsaparilla was included in the *U.S. Pharmacopeia,* and was recommended by the U.S. Dispensatory for the treatment of secondary syphilis. Many people still use sarsaparilla as a tonic today.

POSSIBLE BENEFITS
- Good diuretic—induces sweating and urination.
- Useful for urinary problems.

- Relieves swelling and soreness of arthritis.
- May enhance physical performance.

HOW TO USE IT

Take 1 capsule up to 3 times daily.

Mix 10 to 30 drops of extract in liquid daily. For fevers,
use warm liquid.

SAW PALMETTO

• *Serenoa serrulata* •

FACTS

Recently, a friend told me that he had visited his urologist and, much to his surprise, saw a bottle of saw palmetto on his physician's desk! How times have changed! Just a decade ago, no self-respecting urologist would have told his patients to use this or any other herb. Today, any urologist worth his salt is advising his male patients to take saw palmetto.

Saw palmetto is used to treat benign prostate hypertrophy (BPH), or enlarged prostate. Although the condition is rarely serious, it can be very annoying. In particular, it can cause frequent urination as well as difficulty passing urine, especially at night. This can be as exhausting as it is frustrating. Studies show that saw palmetto is especially effective at relieving urination problems caused by an enlarged prostate. Prescription drugs for BPH also work well, but can have numerous unpleasant side effects, including a sudden drop in blood pressure, which can leave one feeling faint. Although saw palmetto relieves the symptoms associated with BPH, it does not reduce the size of the prostate. The FDA may not recognize saw palmetto as an effective drug, but in Germany it is used in over-the-counter treatments for benign prostate enlargement.

Recently, researchers have begun investigating saw palmetto as a treatment for breast tenderness during menstruation and lactation as well as other women's problems, such as hair loss.

POSSIBLE BENEFITS

- Relieves excessive urination due to benign enlarged prostate.

HOW TO USE IT

Take two 160 mg. capsules daily. (Look for products standardized to contain 85 to 95 percent fatty acids and sterols.)

Personal Advice

This herb works best in combination with nettles, pygeum, zinc, and beta sistosterols, plus soy isoflavones. I take two tablets of this combination twice daily.

> **CAUTION:** Any man who is experiencing pain or swelling of the prostate, or who is having difficulty with urination, or who passes any blood in the urine, should be examined by his physician. Some physicians worry that saw palmetto may mask the symptoms of prostate cancer, in particular producing artificially low PSA (prostate specific antigen) levels. Elevated PSA levels could indicate the presence of cancer. Therefore, it is advisable to be checked by your physician before taking this herb.

SHIITAKE MUSHROOM
• *Lentinus edodes* •

FACTS

These mushrooms contain a polysaccharide called *lentinan,* which has been shown to slow the growth of cancerous tumors in animals. Studies suggest that lentinan may work by enhancing the immune system's ability to fight against infection. This mushroom is used as a cancer-fighting agent in Japan and China. Shiitake also lowers cholesterol, helping to prevent heart disease.

POSSIBLE BENEFITS
- Boosts the immune system.
- Lowers blood cholesterol.

HOW TO USE IT
Take up to 3 capsules daily.

CAUTION: Seek professional advice before using this or any other herb to treat cancer or tumors.

SKULLCAP
• *Scutellaria lateriflora* •

FACTS

As its name implies, the flower of this plant resembles a cap. This herb is known for its calming effect on the body. An antispasmodic, it has been used to relieve menstrual cramps and muscle pain due to stress. It is given to recovering alcoholics suffering from withdrawal symptoms. Also called *mad-dog weed*, skullcap is a traditional remedy for rabies. One old herbal recommends this herb for "explosive headaches of school teachers." Another claims that skullcap soothes excessive sexual desires—this comment was written when this condition was still considered a problem!

POSSIBLE BENEFITS
- Helps reduce nervous tension.
- Good for insomnia.
- Good for muscle tension.

HOW TO USE IT

Take 1 capsule up to 3 times daily.

Mix 1 tablespoon of dried herb with 8 ounces warm
water. Drink 1 cup tea daily.

Mix 3 to 12 drops of extract in liquid daily.

SLIPPERY ELM BARK

• *Ulmus fulva* •

FACTS

There is a high level of mucilage in the bark of this tree, which makes it extremely soothing for scratchy, raw, sore throats and mouth irritations. It is also good for the sore feeling that often follows vomiting. Some herbalists also use it to relieve pain of gastric ulcers.

POSSIBLE BENEFITS

• Provides soothing coating to throat and esophagus.

HOW TO USE IT

Dissolve 1 lozenge in your mouth up to 3 times daily.

SOYBEAN

• *Glycine max* •

The soybean is a legume belonging to the genus *glycine,* which is related to clover, peas, and alfalfa. Known in China as "meat without bones," soybeans have been used for thousands of years as a high-quality, low-cost meat substitute. Soybeans can be made into a bean curd called *tofu,* ground up into soy milk, dehydrated into a high-protein powder, or made into veggie burgers. Although soybeans are a dietary staple in Asia, when the *Herb Bible* was first published in 1992, most Americans considered soybeans to be exotic health food. Today, however, Americans can't get enough soy. Some have incorporated it into their diets, but others are taking soy extract supplements or drinking soy beverages. The soybean explosion is due to recent scientific studies that strongly suggest that soy is a true miracle food. It not only protects against cancer and heart disease, but can even help control menopausal symptoms.

Numerous studies have shown that soy protein can lower high cholesterol. Two ounces (or 50 grams) of soy protein daily can reduce total cholesterol by about 12 percent, and can cut bad LDL cholesterol by about 11 percent.

What is even more compelling is the fact that soybeans appear to reduce the risk of cancer, especially hormone-dependent cancers. In countries where the consumption of soybeans is high, the mortality rate from breast cancer and prostate cancer is significantly lower than that in the United States. Soybeans contain several important cancer-fighting compounds, including *genistein* and *daidzein,* which have been shown to block the growth of prostate-cancer cells and breast-cancer cells in both test-tube and animal studies. Soybeans also contain other hormonelike compounds, called *phytoestrogens,* which block the action of the more potent estrogens in the body that can stimulate the growth of cancerous tumors. In addition, soybeans also are a terrific source of phytic acid and protease inhibitors, two other cancer-fighting compounds.

The phytoestrogens in soy appear to help ease menopausal symptoms. In fact, in Japan, where women eat on average two ounces of soy daily, there is no word for hot flashes, and Japanese women do not seem to suffer the same degree of menopausal discomfort as western women! Many American women who are reluctant to use synthetic hormone-replacement therapy have turned to soy products as estrogen alternatives. These products are sold under the name of soy extract, soy isolate, or soy isoflavones. Some studies suggest that soy can help the body retain calcium, which will help reduce postmenopausal bone loss, which can lead to osteoporosis.

I make it a point to eat soy food daily and take soy isoflavone supplements. I enjoy grilled tofu and vegetables for lunch or a cup of vanilla soy milk as an afternoon snack. If you don't eat soy food regularly, the new soy supplements and beverages make it easier than ever to reap the benefits of soy. I make a soy miracle shake for breakfast, using one scoop of the powder in about 1 cup of nonfat soy milk and 3 ice cubes in a blender. Chocolate or vanilla flavors are my favorite.

POSSIBLE BENEFITS
- Excellent source of low-fat protein.
- Lowers cholesterol.
- Reduces the risk of cancer.
- Eases menopausal symptoms.

HOW TO USE IT

Drink 1 cup soy milk daily with a scoop of vanilla or chocolate-flavored soy food powder (nonfat), or take soy isoflavones in tablets twice daily. Be sure the soy-concentrate supplement contains genistein and daidzein. The usual dose is 10 mg. genistein and daidzein, along with other isoflavones. Fresh green soybeans can be steamed and eaten as a fresh vegetable. Soybean in the pod, known as eda-mame, are quite delicious when cooked.

SPIRULINA

• *Arthrospira platenis* •

FACTS

Spirulina (which means "little spiral") is a single-celled algae found in fresh-water lakes and ponds. It is one of the oldest life forms on earth, producing the oxygen needed for the evolution of other forms of life. Spirulina was a mainstay of the Aztec diet more than five hundred years ago. Biblical scholars speculate that dried spirulina may have been the manna that sustained the Israelites as they wandered through the desert for forty years. Today, spirulina is being touted as a life-giving nutrient, and an excellent source of vitamins, minerals, and essential fatty acids.

Spirulina is rich in iron, potassium, calcium, B vitamins, and protein. It is also packed with *chlorophyll,* the deep-green pigment found in plants that perform photosynthesis. Chlorophyll is an excellent detoxifier, cleansing the body of pollutants and other toxins.

Recent studies show that spirulina is an immune booster that helps the body fight disease. Japanese researchers reported that a carbohydrate found in spirulina could stop the spread of several different types of viruses, including HIV, which causes AIDS; flu; measles; and mumps. An earlier animal study performed in India involved sixty tobacco chewers with precancerous mouth lesions who continued to chew tobacco throughout the study. Forty-five percent of patients who ate 1 gram of spirulina daily showed a complete regression of symptoms as compared to a group of non-spirulina users who experienced only a 7 percent regression rate.

Because it is a source of such high-quality nutrition, spirulina is an excellent supplement for people on weight-loss regimens. It is reputed to cure food cravings and quench the urge for sugary treats.

POSSIBLE BENEFITS
- Good for iron deficient anemia, especially for vegetarians. Excellent source of nutrients.
- Helps bolster immune system.

HOW TO USE IT
Take up to six 500 mg. tablets daily.

SUMA
• *Pfaffia paniculata* •

FACTS

Dubbed "*para todo,*" or "for all things," by Brazilian Indian tribes who first discovered the medicinal uses of this herb, suma is the South American version of ginseng. South of the border, it is used as a tonic.

In North America, it has been used to treat exhaustion resulting from debilitating viral infections such as Epstein-Barr disease, and the mysterious chronic fatigue syndrome.

POSSIBLE BENEFITS
- Energy tonic.
- Fights fatigue.

HOW TO USE IT
Take up to six capsules daily.

Personal Advice
This herb can help perk up people who are recovering from the flu, as well as anyone else who lacks energy and stamina.

TEA-TREE OIL
• *Melaleuca alternifolia* •

FACTS

Tea-tree oil, derived from the tea leaf, is a time-honored remedy for skin problems such as acne, canker sores, insect bites, and nail fungus. Test-tube studies confirm that tea-tree oil is useful against the microorganisms that cause common skin infections. It has also been used to treat vaginal yeast infections. Tea-tree oil is included in skin-care products, shampoos, and even dental floss. You can put a dab of tea-tree oil on a canker sore in your mouth, but it should not be ingested. It may also relieve the discomfort and promote healing of herpes sores.

POSSIBLE BENEFITS
- Helps clear up skin infections.
- Antifungal.

HOW TO USE IT

Apply tea-tree oil preparations directly to problem areas.

> **CAUTION:** Keep away from children—even in small doses it can be toxic to infants and children. This herb should not be taken internally or used by pregnant women. In rare cases, some people may be allergic to tea-tree oil. Apply it to a small area on your skin and wait twenty-four hours to see if it causes an adverse reaction. If nothing happens, you can use it wherever needed.

TURMERIC

• *Circuma longa* •

FACTS

Turmeric is a spice that is a common ingredient in curry powder, in combination with other herbs such as cayenne, garlic, cumin, and onion. Due to its antibacterial properties, turmeric is believed to have been used to preserve food before the widespread use of refrigeration.

Curcumin, a compound extracted from turmeric, is a powerful antioxidant, and is being studied as a potential treatment for skin, breast, and colon cancer. Chinese researchers reported that mice treated with curcumin before being exposed to a potent carcinogen had significantly lower levels of skin cancer than untreated mice. Researchers at Penn State found that curcumin may block the activity of proteins that are essential for the growth of breast tumors.

A natural anti-inflammatory, curcumin is often included in herbal formulas designed to treat the pain and stiffness associated with arthritis.

More than three thousand years ago, Indian healers used turmeric to treat obesity. We now know that turmeric has a beneficial effect on the liver, stimulating the flow of bile and the breakdown of dietary fats. In Asia, turmeric was used to treat stomach disorders, menstrual problems, blood clots, and liver-related ailments, such as jaundice. Modern research performed primarily in Germany and India shows that turmeric protects against gallbladder disease. Herbalists recommend this herb for people with hepatitis C. Studies also confirm that this herb is useful for preventing blood clots and can reduce high cholesterol levels.

POSSIBLE BENEFITS
- Helps prevent sticking together of blood cells that could cause dangerous clots.
- Lowers high cholesterol.
- Good for liver function.
- Helps prevent gallbladder disease.
- Relieves symptoms of arthritis.
- May prevent cancer.

HOW TO USE IT
Take 1 capsule up to 3 times daily.

Personal Advice
A delicious way to get more turmeric in your diet is to eat more curry. The herbs that are combined to make curry help prevent heart disease and stroke by reducing cholesterol and preventing blood clots.

UVA URSI
• Arctostaphylos uva ursi •

FACTS

Also known as *bearberry,* uva ursi's use as a folk remedy for urinary-tract infections has been validated by modern research, which shows that this herb is an effective treatment for bladder and kidney ailments. Uva ursi is also an excellent diuretic.

POSSIBLE BENEFITS
- Relieves pain from cystitis and nephritis.
- Eliminates excessive bloating due to water retention.

HOW TO USE IT
Take up to 3 capsules daily to relieve symptoms.
Mix 1 tablespoon dried herb in 8 ounces warm water.
   Drink 1 cup daily.

VALERIAN
• *Valeriana officinalis* •

FACTS

Dubbed the "Valium of the nineteenth century," valerian, chemically unrelated to the prescription drug Valium, is recognized worldwide for its relaxing effect on the body. In Europe, it is often prescribed to treat anxiety. Unlike many of the prescription drugs commonly used in the United States for this purpose, such as Valium and Xanax, valerian has few unpleasant side effects—other than that it doesn't taste very good—and it is not addictive. Valerian offers another advantage over Valium. Valium has a synergistic effect with alcohol: When taken together, the two drugs greatly exaggerate each other's effect on the body. Not only does this synergistic relationship encourage abuse but, when combined, the two drugs can cause serious side effects. For centuries, valerian has been the treatment of choice by herbalists for nervous tension and panic attacks. It also has been used to relieve muscle cramps related to stress, menstrual cramps, and PMS. Although valerian has been widely studied, how this herb works is still not known.

POSSIBLE BENEFITS
- Has a calming effect.
- Relieves insomnia.

- Good for muscle tension.
- Good for periods of extreme emotional stress.
- Relieves gas pains and stomach cramps.

HOW TO USE IT

Take up to 3 capsules daily to relieve symptoms.
Mix 10 drops of extract in liquid daily.

CAUTION: In extremely high doses, valerian may cause paralysis and a weakening of the heartbeat. Therefore, do not exceed recommended dose. Do not use valerian with other sedatives.

VITEX OR CHASTE TREE
• *Verbenaceae* •

FACTS

In the first edition of the *Herb Bible,* I noted that vitex was an up-and-coming herb, not quite ready for the Hot Hundred, but certainly moving in that direction. Today, vitex has earned a place on the Hot Hundred. Vitex, also known as *chaste tree* and *agnus castus,* is extremely popular in Europe, where it is used to treat PMS as well as some of the unpleasant side effects associated with menopause. In Germany, it has been approved by Commission E for treating the symptoms of menopause. For centuries, this herb has been reputed to be a hormone balancer, and was at one time recommended as a treatment to curb excessive sexual desire. European herbalists use it today to treat fibroid tumors and other women's disorders.

POSSIBLE BENEFITS
- Helps relieve PMS.
- May relieve menopausal symptoms when combined
   with other herbs.

HOW TO USE IT

Take 1 capsule up to 3 times daily.

Mix 20 to 30 drops of extract in liquid up to 3 times daily.

WHITE WILLOW BARK

• *Salix alba* •

FACTS

For centuries, a derivative of this bark, called *salicum,* was used to break fevers, soothe headaches, and reduce pain and swelling in arthritic joints. Based on their studies of salicum, researchers derived a synthetic drug called *acetyl salicylic acid,* better known today as aspirin. Unlike aspirin, which can cause stomach irritation, white willow contains tannins, which are actually good for the digestive system.

POSSIBLE BENEFITS

- Reduces inflammation and fever.
- Relieves pain.
- Good for neuralgia.
- Relieves swollen joints due to rheumatism and arthritis.

HOW TO USE IT

Take 2 capsules every 2 to 3 hours as needed.

Personal Advice

This is an excellent aspirin substitute.

YERBA SANTA

• *Eriodictyon californicum* •

FACTS

The American Indians smoked or chewed the leaves of this plant as a treatment for asthma. It is still used by herbal enthusiasts for bronchial congestion, asthma, and hay fever.

POSSIBLE BENEFITS

- Quiets a nagging cough.
- Helps clear chest of phlegm.
- Relieves congestion due to allergy.

HOW TO USE IT

Mix 1 tablespoon dried herb in 8 ounces warm water. Drink 1 cup daily.
Mix 10 to 20 drops extract in liquid daily.

YOHIMBE

• *Pausinystalia yohimbe* •

FACTS

Yohimbe is extracted from the bark of a tree native to West Africa. A chemical derived from yohimbe, *yohimbine,* is an FDA-approved drug for impotence; it is available by prescription only. Studies have shown that the drug Yohimbine can help between one-third to one-half of men with erection problems. Similar to Viagra, the hot new prescription drug, yohimbine also increases blood flow to the penis. The problem is, yohimbine is not safe for everyone. It can cause a sudden drop in blood pressure and anxiety attacks in some men. The over-the-counter yohimbe products do not cause such serious side effects, but may not be as effective as yohimbine. Yohimbe is often included in herbal products designed to enhance potency, which may also include ginkgo biloba and 1-arginine.

POSSIBLE BENEFITS

- Improves sexual function in men.

HOW TO USE IT

Take up to three 500 mg. capsules daily.

CAUTION: I recommend using this herb under the guidance of a physician or natural healer.

YUCCA

• *Yucca liliaceae* •

FACTS

The Southwestern Indians have used this herb for hundreds of years to treat pain and inflammation of arthritis and rheumatism.

POSSIBLE BENEFITS

- Reduces inflammation.
- Relieves joint pain due to arthritis and rheumatism.

HOW TO USE IT

Take up to 3 tablets or capsules daily to relieve symptoms.

Mix 10 to 30 drops extract in liquid up to 3 times daily.

CAUTION: Long-term use may slow the absorption of fat-soluble vitamins like A, D, E, and K. Check with your health professional to see if supplements of these oil-soluble vitamins are needed if you are using yucca over a period of time.

Reading Between the Lines

The "Doctrine of Signatures," a concept popular in the fifteenth century, espoused that God revealed an herb's medicinal purpose by providing special markings on the plant. There are many herbs that indeed support this theory. For example, the leaves of the lungwort plant, an excellent treatment for upper-respiratory infections and lung ailments, have spotted markings that are characteristic of delicate lung tissue. The root of the ginseng plant, an herb reputed to be good for nearly every organ system, resembles the shape of the human body.

HERBAL TEAS AND THEIR USES

There are two kinds of herbal teas: those that are used primarily as alternative beverages to coffee and regular tea, and those that are valued for their medicinal properties. The former are sold in supermarkets and the herbs are merely used as flavoring agents. These teas are relatively weak and generally harmless, but they do not offer the same benefits of real herbal tea. The real stuff is usually sold in health food stores and herb shops in tea bags or as loose dried herbs. As a rule, these herbal preparations are more potent than the supermarket variety, and should be used more carefully. Before you use any herbal tea, however, you should learn as much as possible about the herb. If you are pregnant or have a medical condition such as high blood pressure, check with your doctor before drinking any herbal tea. Avoid using stimulants such as ephedra at night, or soporific, relaxing herbs such as chamomile early in the day when you may need a lift. Some manufacturers may add caffeine to their packaged herbal products, so if you want to avoid this drug, be sure to read the label very carefully. Your best bet is to buy an herbal tea that is labeled *caffeine-free.*

Making an herbal tea is about as simple as boiling water. Put 1 tablespoon of the herb in a tea ball (infuser) and place in 1 cup of boiling water. Let the mixture steep for five to ten minutes. Remove the tea ball and drink. If you don't want to use a tea ball, simply steep the herbs directly in the hot water and strain after ten minutes. To make several cups at once, use a glass or ceramic tea pot. Use 1 tablespoon of herb for every cup of water. You can sweeten your home-brewed tea with honey.

In warm weather, you can add ice cubes to prepared tea to make your own iced tea. Peppermint, apple, chamomile, cranberry, raspberry, and orange flower are particularly good when chilled. Garnish with lemon or a sprig of fresh mint.

The following is a list of popular herbal teas and a brief description of their reputed uses.

Alfalfa tea	Aids digestion
Angelica tea	Mild antispasmodic and digestive aid
Aniseed tea	Decongestant for nose and sinuses
Basil and borage tea	Pick-me-up tonic
Bilberry tea	Aids circulation
Black currant tea	Stimulates taste buds
Blueberry tea	Pleasant before-meal tea
Borage tea	Combats melancholy
Buchu tea	Natural diuretic (dangerous if taken to excess)
Burdock root tea	Helps sciatica and rheumatoid arthritis
Butcher's broom	Good diuretic
Catnip tea	Relaxant and mild antidepressant
Chamomile tea	Good before bedtime
Chicory tea	Normalizes liver function
Cinnamon tea	Clears the brain and improves thought processes
Cornsilk tea	Reduces pain of urinary infections
Couch grass tea	Good diuretic
Dandelion tea	Improves liver function and kidney function
Elderflower tea	Increases immune function
Fennel tea	Good for the pancreas
Fenugreek tea	Good for colds, clogged ears, and aching sinuses

Ginger tea	Relieves nausea, restores appetite
Ginseng tea	Natural tonic for a mood lift
Goldenseal root tea	Natural antibiotic action
Hawthorne berry tea	Energizing for the elderly
Hops tea	Relaxant and calming agent
Horehound tea	Helps loosen heavy mucus
Jasmine tea	Mild nerve sedative
Juniper berry tea	Helps cystitis or bladder inflammation
Licorice tea	Good laxative
Mate tea	Tones muscles, especially the smooth muscles of the heart
Nettle tea	Increases blood pressure (avoid if you have high blood pressure)
Orange flower tea	Sleep aid
Parsley tea	Diuretic (increases flow of urine)
Peppermint tea	Relieves gas
Raspberry tea	Tightens, tones, and strengthens the uterus
Red clover tea	Relieves menopausal symptoms
Rosehips tea	Adrenal stimulant during daytime
Sage tea	Improves brain nourishment; known as the *thinker's tea*
Sarsaparilla tea	Laxative, hormone balancer, should not be used on a regular basis
Senna tea	Strong laxative
Slippery elm bark	Pain reliever
Spearmint tea	Relieves gas
Thyme	Sore throats and colds
Valerian tea	Natural sedative
Yarrow tea	General tonic

CHAPTER 3

Traditional Favorites

These *time-honored* herbs have been valued for centuries for their reputed medicinal properties, and still have a strong following among traditional herbalists.

ALFALFA

• *Medicago sativa* •

FACTS

First discovered by the Arabs, who dubbed this valuable plant the "father of all foods," the leaves of the alfalfa plant are rich in minerals and nutrients, including calcium, magnesium, potassium, and beta carotene, all of which are useful against both heart disease and cancer. Alfalfa is a good laxative and a natural diuretic, and is often used to treat urinary tract infections. This versatile herb is also a folk remedy for arthritis, and is reputed to be an excellent appetite stimulant and overall tonic. Unfortunately, most westerners regard alfalfa as cattle fodder and, therefore, rarely take advantage of the beneficial properties of this common plant.

POSSIBLE BENEFITS

- Good for cystitis or inflammation of the bladder.
- Boosts a sluggish appetite.
- Provides relief from bloating or water retention.
- Excellent source of nutrients.
- Relieves constipation.
- May reduce swelling and inflammation associated with rheumatism.

HOW TO USE IT

Take 3 to 6 capsules or tablets daily.

Mix 1 tablespoon dried herb with 8 ounces warm water. Drink 1 cup home-brewed tea daily.

Toss alfalfa sprouts in salads.

CAUTION: Alfalfa has been known to aggravate lupus in animal experiments. If you have lupus or other autoimmune problems, avoid this herb.

Personal Advice

For relief from arthritis, take 6 to 9 alfalfa tablets daily.

ANISE

• Pimpinella anisum •

FACTS

Since the era of the ancient Egyptians, sweet-tasting anise seed has been used both as a spice and as a popular remedy. A tea brewed from the crushed seed can relieve digestive disorders and cramps. It also helps loosen phlegm and is useful against coughs and colds. Herbalists recommend anise extract to soothe colicky infants. Since the Middle Ages, anise tea has been sipped by nursing mothers to increase milk production. This old wive's tale appears to be based on fact: A recent study done at Auburn University shows that cows sprayed with anise oil produced more milk than cows sprayed with other fragrances. Recently, scientists discovered that anise contains *phytoestrogens*, plant chemicals similar in structure to the female hormone estrogen. The phytoestrogens in anise may help relieve menopausal symptoms caused by the decline in the body's production of estrogen.

POSSIBLE BENEFITS
- Helps expel gas.
- Promotes digestion.
- Relieves nausea and abdominal pain.
- Soothes coughs and colds, helps clear congestion.
- Stimulates milk production in nursing mothers.
- May reduce menopausal symptoms.

HOW TO USE IT

Crush seeds into powder. Put 1 teaspoon into 1 cup boiling water. Drink up to 3 times daily.

BAYBERRY BARK
• *Myrica certifera* •

FACTS

One of the most versatile herbs, this native American plant is highly regarded by herbal practitioners. Nineteenth-century physicians used to prescribe a hot tea made from the powdered bark of the bayberry at the first sign of a cold, cough, or flu. The tea is an excellent expectorant. It also promotes perspiration, helping you literally to sweat out a cold, and is good for circulation. In large doses, bayberry can induce vomiting, and was, at one time, used to treat cases of poisoning. Bayberry makes an excellent mouthwash, particularly soothing for sore or sensitive gums. Rubbed on the skin, bayberry can be used to reduce the swelling or discomfort caused by varicose veins. It is also one of the oldest remedies for hemorrhoids.

POSSIBLE BENEFITS
- Helps clear congestion in chest due to cold.
- Has a mild stimulating effect.
- Good astringent.
- Soothes inflamed varicose veins.

HOW TO USE IT

Take 1 capsule up to 3 times daily as needed. Mix 10 to 20 drops of extract in juice or water. Gargle with liquid mixture made of extract or powder as needed.

Mix $^1/_2$ to 1 teaspoon of powder in 1 cup warm water. Rub liquid mixture on varicose veins or hemorrhoids as needed.

BLACK WALNUT
• *Juglans nigra* •

FACTS

The fruit, leaves, and bark of this tree offer many benefits. Taken internally, black walnut helps relieve constipation, and is also useful against fungal and parasitic infections. It may also help eliminate warts, which are troublesome growths caused by viruses. Rubbed on the skin, black-walnut extract is reputed to be beneficial for eczema, herpes, psoriasis, and skin parasites.

POSSIBLE BENEFITS
- Fights against fungal infection.
- Antiseptic properties help fight bacterial infection.
- Antiparasitic.
- Helps promote bowel regularity.

HOW TO USE IT

Mix 10 to 20 drops of extract in water or juice daily.
Rub extract on skin 2 times daily.

BLESSED THISTLE

• *Cnicus benedictus* •

FACTS

This herb is one of the oldest folk remedies for the treatment of *amenorrhea,* which is absence of the menstrual cycle after the onset of menstruation. Blessed thistle stimulates the production of bile by the liver, and is often used by folk healers to treat liver disorders. This herb is also reputed to perk up a sluggish appetite, improve circulation, and stimulate memory. Herbalists use blessed thistle to resolve blood clots and to stop bleeding. For menstruation problems, blessed thistle is usually taken in combination with other herbs, such as ginger, cramp bark, and black cohosh root. This herb is often included in commercial herbal preparations designed specifically for women.

POSSIBLE BENEFITS
- Helps regulate menstrual cycle.
- Used in treating liver problems.
- Improves the appetite.
- Lowers fever.
- Helps to stop bleeding.

HOW TO USE IT

Take up to 3 capsules daily.
Mix 10 to 20 drops extract in liquid daily.

CAUTION: Do not use during pregnancy. If you are taking estrogen or birth-control pills, do not use this herb unless under a physician's supervision.

BONESET

• *Eupatorium perfoliatum* •

FACTS

Native Americans introduced the settlers to this New World herb. Its name reflects its use during a particularly harsh strain of flu called *break bone fever*. Come cold and flu season, boneset can be invaluable in relieving coughs and upper-respiratory congestion, helping to loosen up phlegm, and clearing nasal passages. It also can be used to help reduce a fever. This versatile herb has a calming effect on the body and can relieve constipation.

POSSIBLE BENEFITS
- Brings down a fever.
- Relieves flu symptoms.
- Has a calming effect on the body.
- Taken in a warm drink, it is an excellent expectorant.
- Taken in a cold drink, it is a mild laxative.

HOW TO USE IT
Mix 10 to 40 drops extract in liquid daily.

BORAGE

• *Borago officinalis* •

FACTS

In medieval times, borage tea was given to competitors in tournaments as a morale booster. "I, borage, bring always courage," was a popular rhyme of the day. Culpeper noted that this herb can "increase milk in women's breasts," and was excellent for clearing phlegm from the lungs. Through the years, herbalists have used borage to treat a wide range of ailments, from ulcers to frazzled nerves. Borage is also an excellent source of *gamma linoleic acid*, which is used to treat symptoms of PMS.

HOW TO USE IT

This herb is available in extract and capsules. Take up to 3 capsules daily. Mix 1 teaspoon of extract in juice. Drink daily.

BUCHU

• *Barosma betulina* •

FACTS

Almost four hundred years ago, the Hottentots, a native tribe of South Africa, recognized the many healing properties of this aromatic plant. Combined with the Hot Hundred herb uva ursi, buchu is best known as a remedy for urinary disorders including cystitis and prostate-related problems. It also helps reduce bloating and excess water weight and promotes perspiration.

POSSIBLE BENEFITS
- Useful for urinary tract infections.
- Good diuretic.
- Has a stimulating effect on the body.

HOW TO USE IT
Take up to 3 capsules daily.
Mix 10 to 30 drops of extract in juice or water.

CAUTION: Do not use for kidney infections or if you have any kidney problems, since buchu can be irritating to the kidneys. Kidney infections need prompt medical attention. If you have pain during urination, or blood in the urine, call your doctor immediately.

The Marijuana Story

Cannabis, the dried, flowering spikes of the hemp plant, is a well-known psychoactive drug that was made into hashish by certain Muslim sects in the Middle Ages. The word *assassin* is derived from the Arab *hashshashin,* which refers to a secret order of Muslim that terrorized the Christian crusaders by committing murder while under the influence of this potent drug.

CARAWAY

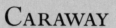

• *Carum carvi* •

FACTS

The seeds from this plant, which are often used in baked goods, are known for their mildly spicy, aromatic flavor. Caraway is soothing for gas and other stomach disorders. It can also increase the appetite. Brewed into a tea, the warm fluid is excellent for coughs and colds. For centuries, midwives have used caraway extract to stimulate the production of breast milk in nursing mothers, and to ease colic in infants.

POSSIBLE BENEFITS

- Excellent digestive aid.
- Helps expel gas.
- Reduces nausea.
- Improves the appetite.
- Works as an effective expectorant for coughs due to colds.
- Increases breast milk in nursing mothers.

HOW TO USE IT

Mix 3 to 4 drops extract in liquid, 3 to 4 times daily.

For colic, mix 1 to 2 drops in infant formula for 2 feedings. Check with your pediatrician before giving this or any other herb to your baby or child.

Chew the seeds 3 to 4 times daily.

CAUTION: Never give seeds to infants or young children; stick to the extract.

CARDAMOM

• *Elletaria cardamomum* •

FACTS

Grown in India, these pungent, aromatic seeds contain a large amount of a volatile oil that helps stimulate digestion and relieve gas. A mild stimulant, cardamom is a standard ingredient in curry.

HOW TO USE IT

For indigestion, mix 15 crushed seeds in $1/2$ cup hot water. Add 1 ounce fresh ginger root and a cinnamon stick. Simmer 15 minutes over low heat. Add $1/2$ cup milk and simmer 10 more minutes. Add 2 to 3 drops vanilla. Sweeten with honey. Drink 1 to 2 cups daily.

CASCARA SAGRADA OR BUCKTHORN

• *Rhamnus purshiana* •

FACTS

Cascara, also called *buckthorn,* works by stimulating the lining of the upper intestines to promote normal bowel function. It is one of nature's milder laxatives and is effective against chronic constipation.

POSSIBLE BENEFITS

• Relieves constipation overnight.

HOW TO USE IT

Take 1 to 3 capsules or tablets daily.

CAUTION: Excessive dose can cause cramps and diarrhea. Do not use during pregnancy.

Personal Advice

In my many years as pharmacist, I have found that the bark from the California buckthorn is still the most effective laxative known.

CATNIP

• *Nepeta cataria* •

FACTS

This herb is well known for its ability to drive felines into a frenzy, but it actually has the opposite effect on humans. Catnip is a mild sedative that is useful for cramps and upset stomach. In Europe, this herb is a popular remedy for bronchitis and diarrhea. Catnip promotes sweating and has a warming effect on the body.

POSSIBLE BENEFITS
- Helps you relax.
- Eases indigestion and gas.
- May help relieve bronchitis.
- Helps control diarrhea.

HOW TO USE IT
Take 1 to 3 capsules daily.
Mix $^1/_2$ to 1 teaspoon in $^1/_2$ cup warm water and drink.

CHICKWEED

• *Stellaria media* •

FACTS

Culpeper wrote that chickweed "boiled with hog's grease applied, helpeth cramps, convulsions and palsy." In folk medicine, this herb has been used as an expectorant and an antacid. Used externally in ointment form, it is reputed to be excellent for bruises, irritations, eczema, and other skin problems.

HOW TO USE IT

Take 1 capsule up to 3 times daily. Use ointment as needed.

CHIVES

• *Allium schoenoprasum* •

FACTS

High in vitamin C and iron, these members of the lily family can easily be grown at home in a window box, or can be found fresh at most greengrocers or supermarkets. *Allium* vegetables, which include chives, onions and garlic, contain natural cancer-fighting compounds. Chives are reputed to stimulate the appetite and aid in digestion. High in iron, they are useful against anemia. First discovered in China five thousand years ago, chives later became popular in Europe, not only for their subtle onion flavor, but because of the widespread belief that their grasslike leaves could chase away evil spirits and disease. It was not uncommon to find clusters of chives hanging from ceilings and bedposts.

POSSIBLE BENEFITS

- Good for the digestion.
- Helps prevent anemia caused by iron deficiency.

HOW TO USE IT

Chop and sprinkle on salads or other food.

Personal Advice

In order to receive maximum benefit, chives must be eaten fresh. This is one herb that you can even grow at home!

CLOVES
• *Caryophyllum aromaticus* •

FACTS

Cloves are actually the dried buds of the clove tree. Used in China for more than two thousand years, legend has it that cloves are an aphrodisiac. Although there isn't any evidence to back up this claim, we do know that oil of clove is a time-honored remedy for toothache. Clove oil is highly antiseptic. It is also used to stop vomiting.

POSSIBLE BENEFITS
- Relieves tooth pain.
- Has an antiemetic action that helps control vomiting.

HOW TO USE IT
For toothache, rub oil on affected area.
For vomiting, mix 2 drops of oil in a cup of water.

CUCUMBER
• *Cucumis sativus* •

FACTS

Since ancient times, the juice of the cucumber has been used as a facial cleanser and as a treatment for skin irritations. Cleopatra herself was reputed to have used cucumber to preserve her beautiful skin. Culpeper recommends cucumber to ease sunburn and to lighten freckles. Eaten as a vegetable, cucumber is a good diuretic and can help prevent constipation. Researchers are now investigating an extract of cucumber as a possible cholesterol buster.

HOW TO USE IT

Place cucumber slices on irritated areas. Eat the fresh vegetable. Cucumber juice is also used in many skin products.

DAMIANA

• *Turnera aphrodisiaca* •

FACTS

As its botanical name suggests, damiana is reputed to be a sexual stimulant and folk cure for impotence. This herb is also put to more mundane uses: Herbalists recommend it as both a laxative and as a general tonic to improve overall body function. Some herbalists believe that it helps relieve anxiety and promotes a feeling of well-being.

POSSIBLE BENEFITS

- May enhance sexual performance.
- Helps relieve constipation.
- May create a good mood!

HOW TO USE IT

Take up to 3 capsules daily before meals.
Mix 10 to 30 drops extract in liquid daily.

DILL

• *Aniethum graveolens* •

FACTS

Since biblical times, dill has been cultivated for its aromatic seeds. Widely used in cooking, dill is best known as a digestive aid and remedy for a sour, gassy stomach. It is also used to promote milk production in nursing mothers. Chewing dill seed is an old-time cure for bad breath.

POSSIBLE BENEFITS

- Soothes indigestion and upset stomach.
- Promotes appetite.
- Helps milk production in nursing mothers.
- Helps expel gas.

HOW TO USE IT

Steep 2 teaspoons dill seed in 1 cup water for 10 to 15 minutes. Strain. Drink up to 3 cups daily.

ELECAMPANE

• *Inula helenium* •

FACTS

This herb is a traditional remedy for respiratory-tract infections and digestive problems. It is not only a good expectorant, its essential oils and high mucilage content provide a soothing, protective coating that can relieve irritation due to excessive coughing. Culpeper endorsed elecampane wholeheartedly: "It has not its equal in the cure of whooping-cough in children, when all other medicines fail." Once held in high regard by the medical establishment, this herb was listed in the *U.S. Pharmacopeia*. Elecampane was also a folk cure for amenorrhea, or loss of menstruation. This or any other herb that can induce menstruation should not be used during pregnancy.

HOW TO USE IT

Use the dried herb to make tea. Drink 1 cup daily. Mix 10 to 30 drops of extract in liquid. Drink up to 3 times daily.

EUCALYPTUS

• *Eucalyptus globulus* •

FACTS

Koala bears eat them, but human beings, too, have relied on the leaves of this plant for a wide range of medicinal purposes. The oil of eucalyptus and its active ingredient, *eucalyptol,* are frequently found in over-the-counter cough drops and salves. The oil is also commonly used in steam-inhalation preparations for colds and flu: A few whiffs is often all it takes to clear a stuffy nose and a foggy head. Rubbed on the skin, eucalyptus oil provides relief from the pain of arthritis and rheumatism. It increases blood flow to the area, thus producing a feeling of warmth. When aged, the oil forms *ozone,* a form of oxygen that specifically destroys bacteria, fungi, and viruses.

POSSIBLE BENEFITS

- Helps relieve upper respiratory distress caused by cold and flu.
- Good expectorant.
- Good antiseptic.
- Can help soothe stiffness and swelling of arthritis and rheumatism.

HOW TO USE IT

Put 1 to 5 drops of extract in a vaporizer. Use liniment as needed.

CAUTION: Do not use on broken or irritated skin. Do not use internally.

Personal Advice
Currently, a widely advertised commercial rub contains eucalyptus and mint together in an ointment for arthritis.

Hops
• *Humulus lupulus* •

FACTS

Despite its name, hops has a calming effect on the body. It is used to relieve gas and cramps—it soothes muscle spasms—and can stimulate the appetite. Hops was originally used in ale as a preservative. For an old-time cure for insomnia, sprinkle hops with alcohol, put it in a pillowcase, and sleep on it.

POSSIBLE BENEFITS
- Has a calming effect.
- Relieves indigestion.
- An old-time pain reliever.
- A good after-dinner tea.

HOW TO USE IT
Take up to 3 capsules daily.
Mix 1 teaspoon of dried herb in $1/2$ cup warm water.
Drink 1 cup daily.

Just Wild About Saffron?

Saffron is the world's most expensive spice. It retails for more than forty dollars an ounce, and no wonder. It takes 50,000 *stigmas*—a small part of the pistil of the flower—to make a mere 4 ounces of this precious spice. At one time, it was highly regarded for its medicinal properties. In 1597, English herbalist John Gerard wrote, "For those at death's doure and almost past breathing, saffron bringeth breath again." Today, saffron is used primarily in cooking—by those who can afford it.

HOREHOUND

• *Marrubium vulgare* •

FACTS

This is the herb to keep on hand when you have a bad cough due to a cold or bronchitis. It is not only an excellent expectorant but it promotes sweating, which can help break a fever. A mild stimulant, horehound can help relieve the dragged-out, sluggish feeling that often accompanies a bad cold. It is also good for the digestion.

POSSIBLE BENEFITS
- Relieves symptoms of coughs and colds.
- Rids body of excess water weight.
- Promotes sweating, helps cool off the body.

HOW TO USE IT
For coughs, mix 10 to 40 drops of extract in warm water. Use up to 3 times daily.

Horehound drops (candy lozenges) can be used to soothe the throat.

HORSERADISH

• *Armoracia lapathifolia* •

FACTS

The flavor of the horseradish root is so bitter that it brings tears to the eyes, which is why it is included in the traditional Passover meal to commemorate the suffering of the Jews under the Pharaoh's rule. It is also an excellent diuretic and good for digestion. Herbalists combine horseradish with honey for coughs and asthma. Externally, it can be used to alleviate the pain and stiffness caused by rheumatism.

POSSIBLE BENEFITS
- Good expectorant, soothing for respiratory problems.
- May help relieve rheumatism by stimulating blood flow to inflamed joints.

HOW TO USE IT
Mix grated root with honey and warm water. Use daily for bad cough. It may not taste very good, but it is very effective.

Tablets are available in Australia. Use as directed.

Fresh horseradish can be made into a poultice by adding it to cornstarch. Apply to affected areas in a gauze bandage.

CAUTION: Do not consume large quantities at one time—it may cause diarrhea and excessive sweating.

Personal Advice
It's best to use the fresh product if it is available at your grocery store or herb store.

HORSETAIL
• *Equisetum arvense* •

FACTS

Long used by herbal healers in Europe and China, horsetail—also known as *silica*—is rich in nutrients, including silicon. Horsetail facilitates the absorption of calcium by the body, which nourishes nails, skin, hair, bones, and the body's connective tissue. This herb helps eliminate excess oil from skin and hair, and is believed to make individual hair strands stronger, thicker, and more resilient.

POSSIBLE BENEFITS
- Good conditioner for nails and hair.
- Helps eliminate white spots from nails.
- Controls excess oil on skin.
- Helps strengthen bones.

HOW TO USE IT
Take up to 3 capsules daily.
Horsetail is used in many herbal beauty products for
    skin, nails, and hair.

HYSSOP
• *Hyssopus officinalis* •

FACTS

This herb is useful in treating a bad cold's cough and stuffy nose. It will help relieve the heavy, congested feeling in the head and chest. Studies show that it has antiviral properties and can be useful in treating cold sores. It can also be used for indigestion.

POSSIBLE BENEFITS
- Good expectorant for coughs and cold.
- Relieves gas.
- Improves the appetite.
- Good gargle for sore throat.

HOW TO USE IT

Mix 1 teaspoon of dried herb in $^1/_2$ cup warm water.
Drink up to 3 times daily for cough.
Gargle up to 3 times daily for sore throats and cold
sores.
Take 1 to 2 teaspoons of extract daily.
Dissolve one lozenge in the mouth as needed to soothe a
sore throat.

CAUTION: Do not take for more than two weeks without seeking medical advice.

ICELAND MOSS
• *Centraria islandica* •

FACTS

This plant is not a moss at all, but a plant form called a *lichen,* which is made up of fungus and algae. Still used to treat tuberculosis in some parts of the world, Iceland moss is a folk remedy for coughs and congestion due to colds.

HOW TO USE IT

Use the dried herb to make tea. Mix 1 teaspoon of the
herb in $^1/_2$ cup hot water daily. For best results,
sip slowly. Use this herb only to treat specific

symptoms. Do not use it for more than two weeks at a time.

JASMINE

• *Jasminum officinale*

FACTS

For centuries, the flowers from the jasmine plant have been brewed into a tea that is both delicious and relaxing. Many commercial jasmine teas are available today. According to folklore, the oil from this flower can be sexually arousing if rubbed on the body.

POSSIBLE BENEFITS
- Has a calming effect.
- Good after-dinner drink.
- Possible aphrodisiac.

HOW TO USE IT
Drink 1 cup of tea daily.

JUNIPER BERRY

• *Juniperus communis* •

FACTS

In the 1500s, a Dutch pharmacist used juniper berry to create a new, inexpensive diuretic that he called *gin.* The drink caught on for other reasons, and the juniper berry is now just one of several ingredients. For centuries, juniper has been a folk remedy for urinary-tract problems, including urinary retention and gallstones. It has also been used successfully to treat *gout,* a condition marked by painful inflammation of the joints caused by deposits of uric acid and high uric-acid content in the blood. The berry is good for digestion and can help eliminate gas and cramps.

POSSIBLE BENEFITS
- Relieves urinary tract problems.
- Old-time treatment for gout.
- Helps improve digestion.
- Helps rid the body of excess fluid.

HOW TO USE IT
Take 10 to 20 drops extract up to 3 times daily.
Drink 1 cup tea up to 3 times daily.

CAUTION: Do not use during pregnancy.

LADY'S MANTLE
• *Alchemilla vulgaris* •

FACTS

Women in Arab countries believe that this herb restores beauty and youth—needless to say, it is very popular in that part of the world. Traditionally, lady's mantle has been used by Western herbalists topically on wounds to stop bleeding and promote healing. Taken internally, it is used to regulate menstruation and stimulate the appetite. It also makes a soothing douche for mild vaginal irritations. The botanical name, *alchemilla*, is derived from the word *alchemy*, because the herbs in this family are believed to bring about miraculous cures.

POSSIBLE BENEFITS
- Promotes coagulation of blood, stops bleeding.
- Promotes menstrual regularity.
- Improves appetite.
- Reduces vaginal irritation.

HOW TO USE IT

Put 1 tablespoon of dried herb in hot water. Drink 1
cup daily.

Dissolve 5 to 10 drops of extract in 16 ounces of water
and use as a douche. It can also be applied to
wounds.

LEMON BALM
• *Melissa officinalis* •

FACTS

This tea was originally grown in the Orient; Arab traders later introduced this herb to Spain. It was later brought to Germany by Benedic-
tine monks. Still popular in Europe, lemon balm is now grown in parts
of the United States. A member of the mint family, lemon balm contains volatile oils, which provide its pleasant, lemony scent. This herb
has long been a folk remedy for gas and colic. The famous seventeenth-
century herbalist Culpeper thought so highly of lemon balm that he
wrote, "Let a syrup made with the juice of it and sugar . . . be kept in
every gentle woman's house to relieve the weak stomachs and sick bodies of their poor and sickly neighbours." Herbalists still prescribe this
herb for upset stomach, nervous tension, and insomnia. A mild di-
aphoretic, lemon balm induces sweating when taken hot. This cools the
body and can help break a fever.

A recent study reported that a cream derived from lemon balm extract is extremely effective in treating *herpes simplex labialis,* which
causes cold sores around the mouth.

HOW TO USE IT

This herb is widely available in tea, dried herb, extract, and creams for external use. Mix $1/2$ to 1 teaspoon of extract in liquid up to 3 times daily. Use the dried herb to make tea, or drink 1 cup of packaged tea daily. Use external creams as directed.

LUNGWORT

• *Pulmonaria officinalis* •

FACTS

As its name suggests, this herb is good for coughs, hoarseness, and mild lung problems. It can also be used for diarrhea, which makes it the herb of choice for a stomach virus accompanied by a cough.

POSSIBLE BENEFITS

• Good expectorant, breaks up chest congestion.
• Can soothe throat irritation.
• Helps cure diarrhea.

HOW TO USE IT

Mix 1 tablespoon of dried herb in 1 cup hot water. Drink 1 cup daily.

CAUTION: If you have a cough that lasts for more than two weeks, do not try to self-medicate. See a medical professional immediately.

MEADOWSWEET

• *Filipendula ulmaria* •

FACTS

This herb was reputed to be the favorite of Queen Elizabeth I because of its sweet, fragrant scent. Long a remedy for flu, fever, and arthritis, meadowsweet contains an aspirin-type compound called *salicylic acid*. The tea is regarded as an excellent diuretic.

HOW TO USE IT

Make tea from the dried herb. Drink 1 cup daily.

MOTHERWORT

• *Leonurus cardiaca* •

FACTS

Since ancient times, this herb has been used both to treat "women's disorders" and as a cardiotonic. The Greeks used motherwort to relieve the pain from childbirth and as a tranquilizer. Culpeper wrote, "There is no better herb to take melancholy vapours from the heart and to strengthen it." Modern herbalists use motherwort to treat PMS.

HOW TO USE IT

Mix 10 to 15 drops extract in warm liquid up to 3 times daily.
Use dried herb to make tea. Drink 1 cup daily.

CAUTION: Do not use during pregnancy.

Mullein

• *Verbascum thapsus* •

FACTS

This herb is an old-time remedy for bronchitis and dry, unproductive coughs. It is a good expectorant and, in the process of clearing out congestion, it also soothes irritation in the throat and bronchial passages. An antispasmodic, mullein can relieve stomach cramps and help control diarrhea.

POSSIBLE BENEFITS

- Reduces irritation due to coughs and bronchitis.
- Helps relieve gastrointestinal stress.

HOW TO USE IT

Mix 1 tablespoon dried herb in 8 ounces warm water.
Drink 1 to 2 cups tea daily.
Mix 25 to 40 drops extract in liquid. Drink 3 to 4 times
daily for coughs.

Personal Advice

This is a good herb to have handy for a flu accompanied by stomach cramps, or a chest cold. For those of you who can find the actual plant, the leaves can be boiled in water and the steam can be inhaled to relieve coughs and congestion.

MUSTARD (WHITE AND BLACK)

• *Brassica hirta, Brassica nigra* •

FACTS

Both varieties of mustard plant have similar properties, although black mustard is regarded as the stronger of the two. Culpeper recommended that mustard be used externally for joint pain and backache and be taken internally with honey for coughs. Through the years, herbalists have pretty much followed his advice. Today, however, mustard is usually used externally.

HOW TO USE IT

Mustard oil diluted with rubbing alcohol can be applied to the skin to increase the flow of blood to arthritic areas. Never use the undiluted oil; it can be very irritating. When I was a child, my mother used to apply a mustard plaster to my chest when I had a bad cold—the warming action of the mustard was very soothing. The plaster is easy to make with prepared mustard powder. Mix cold water with the powder to make a thick paste. Spread the paste on a clean cloth and put a layer of gauze over the mustard. Apply to the chest or to arthritic joints. Remove after 10 minutes. Prolonged use can result in skin irritation. The leaves of the white mustard plant can be used in salad and are quite tasty.

MYRRH

• *Commiphora myrrha* •

And when they came into the house, they saw the young child with Mary his mother, and fell down, and worshiped him: and when they had opened their treasures, they presented unto him gifts; gold, and frankincense, and myrrh.

—MATTHEW 2:11

FACTS

Since ancient times, the resin or gum of the myrrh plant has been used as a mouthwash for sores in the mouth and throat. It is also a popular treatment for irritated and infected gums. In addition, myrrh may help relieve upper-respiratory infections due to coughs and cold. It not only soothes irritated bronchial passages, but studies also suggest that myrrh stimulates the body's immune system, increasing resistance to infection. According to the Bible, both Kings David and Solomon sang the praises of this herb, which was also used by Moses in Jewish ceremonial rites. Myrrh was so highly regarded, according to scripture, that it was presented to the infant Jesus by the three wise men.

POSSIBLE BENEFITS
- Excellent antiseptic and mouthwash.
- Promotes healing of mouth sores.
- Strengthens "spongy" or soft gums.
- Good for coughs and colds.
- Good for stomach flu.

HOW TO USE IT
Mix 1 tablespoon dried herb to 8 ounces warm water.
    Drink 1 cup tea daily for colds.
Mix 2 to 5 drops extract in water for an excellent
    mouthwash.

CAUTION: Very high doses over a long period of time can be dangerous. Therefore, do not exceed recommended dose. Do not use if you are pregnant or have kidney disease without first checking with your physician.

PENNYROYAL

• *Hedeoma pulegioides* •

FACTS

Often referred to as the *lung mint,* this herb was used to treat coughs and colds. It promotes perspiration, which helps break a fever. American Indians used pennyroyal to relieve menstrual cramps. Herbalists use pennyroyal today to induce menstruation and to treat monthly symptoms associated with premenstrual syndrome, such as bloating and breast tenderness.

POSSIBLE BENEFITS
- Helps promote productive cough.
- Brings on menstruation.
- Relieves PMS and menstrual cramps.

HOW TO USE IT
Mix 1 tablespoon dried herb with 8 ounces warm water and take daily.

Mix 20 to 40 drops of extract in liquid daily for relief of symptoms.

CAUTION: Back in the days when abortion was illegal, this herb was used to induce abortion. In some cases, it resulted in hemorrhaging and serious complications for the mother. Therefore, it should never be used for this purpose. Today, pennyroyal is one of the herbs used by herbalists to facilitate labor and delivery. **It should be used only under the supervision of a knowledgeable practitioner.** If you do use this herb, do not exceed the recommended dose and do not take for more than a week at a time. In excess, it can cause liver damage.

PLEURISY ROOT
• *Asclepias tuberosa* •

FACTS

As its name suggests, this herb is used for ailments involving the lungs and upper-respiratory problems. It's also good for indigestion and gassy stomach. Native Americans used this root to treat bronchitis, pneumonia, and diarrhea.

POSSIBLE BENEFITS
- Helps clear phlegm from chest.
- Good digestive aid.

HOW TO USE IT
Mix 1 tablespoon dried herb with 8 ounces warm liquid. Drink 1 cup daily.
Mix 5 to 40 drops extract in liquid every 3 hours for relief of symptoms.

CAUTION: The fresh root can be dangerous. Use only commercial preparations.

SAGE

• *Salvia officinalis* •

FACTS

This herb's botanical name is derived from the Latin *salvere,* which means to save, a testimony to sage's early reputation as a cure-all. In the Middle Ages, sage was used to prevent the night sweats typical of tuberculosis patients. Herbalists still recommend it for people who suffer from excessive perspiration. Culpeper prescribed sage tea as a mouthwash for sore gums. The tea is also used for stomach cramps and gas. A popular cooking herb, sage is reputed to be good for the digestion.

HOW TO USE IT

Make a tea from the dried herb. Drink daily. Use tea as a gargle for sore gums up to 3 times daily. Use this delicious herb in your cooking.

THYME

• *Thymus vulgaris* •

FACTS

In the Middle Ages, thyme was believed to increase courage: Women would give a sprig of thyme to their favorite knights before they went into battle. Culpeper wrote that thyme was "a strengthener of the lungs," and "taken internally, comforts the stomach much, and expels wind." Through the years, thyme has been used as an expectorant and a disinfectant and is known for its antifungal properties. It also makes a good gargle for sore throats.

HOW TO USE IT

> Make tea from the dried herb. Drink daily, or gargle
> with it up to 3 times daily. Rub extract between
> toes for athlete's foot daily. The extract can also be
> applied externally for crabs, lice, and scabies. Use
> daily.

WILD OREGON GRAPE

• *Mahonia aquifolium* •

FACTS

Native to North America, this herb became popular in Europe as a
"blood purifier." Wild Oregon grape is believed to enhance liver function and is used to treat jaundice, hepatitis, and other liver ailments. It
is also reputed to be good for eczema and psoriasis. This herb is also
used as a diuretic, and is widely available in extract and dried herb.

HOW TO USE IT

> Make tea from dried herb. Drink daily. Mix 10 to 30
> drops of extract in liquid daily.

WITCH HAZEL

• *Hamamelis virginiana* •

FACTS

First used by North America Indians, witch hazel is an essential item for
every home medicine cabinet. Available in liquid extract, witch hazel's
anti-inflammatory action is very soothing for minor scrapes, cuts, and
bruises. Applied directly to hemorrhoids and varicose veins, it helps re-

lieve the pain and inflammation typical of these conditions. Splashed on the face, it is a revitalizing skin tonic that helps eliminate excess oil.

HOW TO USE IT

Apply factory-distilled extract to irritated areas several
times daily.

HERBS IN THE BIBLE

And God said,"Let the earth bring
forth grass, the herb yielding seed, and the fruit tree yielding
fruit after his kind, whose seed is in itself
upon the earth: and it was so."

—GENESIS 1:11

Throughout the Old and New Testaments—from the Garden of Eden through the Gospels—there are numerous references to herbs that were commonly used in biblical times. The Fertile Crescent, one of the earliest centers of civilization, was full of orchards, woods, and lush, tropical vegetation. The first man, Adam, was a gardener and his son, Cain, grew vegetables. Our ancestors literally lived off the land and, as a result, had a great respect for nature. The ancient Hebrews believed that nature was a gift from God and held His creation in very high esteem.

Herbs such as cinnamon, pomegranate bark, aloe, garlic, onions, cloves, and saffron are frequently mentioned throughout the Bible. On at least one occasion, an herb actually plays an important role in the story line. In Genesis, Leah and Rachel, both wives of Jacob, were constantly vying for his favor. Leah had conceived many sons for Jacob, but Rachel had remained barren. When Leah's son Reuben finds a *mandrake,* a reputed aphrodisiac, Rachel pleads with Leah to give it to her. In exchange for the precious fruit, Rachel agrees to let Leah spend the night with Jacob. Leah promptly conceives another child, but later, so does Rachel. To this day, mandrakes are called "love apples" in the Middle East, and are still valued for their supposed aphrodisiac qualities.

The ancient Hebrews apparently had a healthy reverence for plant medicines. In Ecclesiastes, we are told, "The Lord created medicines from the earth, and a sensible man doesn't despise them."

The Bible also forbids short-term exploitation of the land, a rule that future generations have chosen to ignore. For example, in Leviticus, there are many laws concerning the preservation of trees. God says, "Thou shalt not destroy the trees thereof by forcing an axe against them: for thou may eatest of them, and thou shalt not cut them down for the tree of the field is man's life."

CHAPTER 4

Herbs from Around the World

S*ince the first* edition of the *Herb Bible,* the biggest change in herbal medicine has been the explosive growth of the foreign herb market in the United States. When I first wrote this chapter, foreign herbs were primarily available in tiny hole-in-the-wall shops in ethnic neighborhoods. Each shopkeeper played the role of the village shaman. A customer would describe his or her complaint or a problem to the shopkeeper, who would then fill a bag with a mysterious blend of dried roots, seeds, and leaves. There was simply no way of knowing the potency of these herbs or, for that matter, precisely what was in the mix. Needless to say, a lot was taken on faith. Surprisingly, many of these shopkeeper/herbalists were quite knowledgeable and did a remarkable repeat business. But, like the milkman and the corner five-and-dime, those small herb shops are fast disappearing. Of course, there are still some botanicas selling South American herbs in Latin American neighborhoods, and Chinese herb shops in the Chinatowns of big cities, but they are few and far between. They are being replaced by the slick, modern, natural food stores and pharmacies selling the same herbs once sold in these quaint herbal shops, only in prepackaged, standardized extract forms. Although to some diehard herbalists, buying standardized herbs may be the equivalent of fast food, the reality is that it is now easier than ever for people to use foreign herbs. More than anything else, it has added an international flavor to the practice of herbalism.

Nearly every culture has developed its own style of herbal medicine. Although many rely on the same herbs, each nationality has left its own unique imprint on this universal healing system. In this chapter, I focus on four different forms of herbal healing that I feel have greatly influenced the practice of herbal medicine today: the Ayurvedic form of traditional medicine in India, traditional Chinese medicine, South American medicine, and Native American medicine. Herbs that are also included in the Hot Hundred are designated by an asterisk. See Hot Hundred entries for more information.

▪ Ayurveda: The Traditional Medicine of India

When I first wrote the *Herb Bible,* Ayurvedic herbs, the traditional herbal medicine of India, were considered by westerners to be exotic at best, and weird at worst. In the blink of an eye, these herbs have become integrated into western culture. For this, we owe a debt of gratitude to Deepek Chopra, the physician and healer who popularized Ayurvedic herbs in his books. These herbs have become so popular that several are now sold in discount drug stores and even supermarkets!

More than five thousand years old, the traditional herbal medicine of India may be the oldest healing system in the world. Ayurveda is believed to have provided the foundation of many other healing systems, including traditional Chinese medicine, Tibetan medicine, and the medicine of ancient Greece. It's interesting to note that we credit Greek physician Hippocrates with being the father of modern medicine, yet much of what he advocated can be found in the Ayurveda! Hippocrates is believed to have said, "Let food be your medicine and medicine be your food," yet this is fundamental to Ayurveda, which incorporates food and lifestyle into its approach.

Ayurveda is the combination of two Sanskrit words: *ayu,* which means life, and *veda,* which means knowledge. According to Indian folklore, this precious knowledge was passed down from the Creator, known as *Brahma.* Similar to the ancient Roman and Greek theories of medicine, Ayurveda classified herbs according to five elements: earth, water, fire, air, and ether. Herbs also were subdivided according to five tastes: sweet, sour, salty, pungent, bitter, and astringent. Ayurveda emphasizes health through the pursuit of physical, mental, and spiritual health. In many ways, Ayurveda was ahead of its time: It does not focus on treating illness. It places as much importance on diet and lifestyle as it does on medicinal cures, a philosophy that twentieth-century physicians are finally beginning to accept.

Ayurveda is still widely practiced in India today. The message of Ayurveda is a simple one and best summed up by the following Indian saying: "May everyone be happy. May everyone be healthy. May everyone be holy. May there never be disharmony of any kind, anywhere."

Herbs used in Ayurveda include many of the same herbs that are popular in the West, including alfalfa, aloe vera, devil's claw, echinacea, goldenseal, licorice root, fennel, fenugreek, and turmeric, all Hot Hundred herbs. Ayurveda also includes some exotic herbs that are just being discovered by the West. The following is a list of commonly used Ayurvedic herbs. Since these herbs have not been well researched in the West, I would not recommend using them unless under the supervision of a knowledgeable practitioner.

Popular Ayurvedic Herbs

AMALAKI
• *Phyllanthus emblica* •

FACTS

For thousands of years, this herb has been used to treat coughs and eating disorders, and to normalize bowel function. It is also used to treat skin diseases and tumors. Rich in vitamin C, this herb is included in many Ayurvedic formulas designed to boost immune function.

ASHWAGANDHA*

• *Withania somniforal* •

FACTS

This herb is a true tonic, in that it is used to promote overall health and well being. Often called *Indian ginseng,* it is now one of the most popular of the Ayurvedic herbs. Ashwaganda, a natural anti-inflammatory, is believed to protect the body from the harmful effects of stress. Ancient practitioners of the Ayurvedic used it to promote the healing of broken bones. Ashwangandha is available in capsules and in combination formulas designed to revitalize the body.

BRAHMI OR GOTU KOLA*

• *Hydrocotyle asiatica* •

FACTS

Brahmi is used to relieve anxiety and also as a treatment for epilepsy and leprosy. A natural tranquilizer that has a mild calming effect, brahmi is a popular treatment for skin ailments, such as psoriasis, which are known to be aggravated by stress.

COLEUS FORSKOHLII

FACTS

This herb is an ancient remedy for high blood pressure that is now incorporated in special formulas designed to reduce blood pressure. Indian physicians use this herb to treat heart failure and angina. Use this herb under the supervision of a knowledgeable physician or healer.

GUDUCHI

• *Tinospora cordifolia* •

FACTS

This herb is a diuretic that can lower high blood pressure. Although it is now sold over the counter, if you have high blood pressure, you should use this or any other natural treatment only under the supervision of a qualified practitioner.

GUGGULIPID*

• *Cammiphora mukul* •

FACTS

This Hot Hundred herb is a traditional remedy for "bad" blood lipids. It lowers total cholesterol and triglycerides but raises good HDLs. It is widely available in capsule form. It may also stimulate thyroid function, which would speed up metabolic function.

GYMNEMA SYLVESTRE

FACTS

Known as the *sugar killer*, gynema sylvestre has been used to treat diabetes. It is also reputed to curb the desire for sweets. Ayurvedic healers recommend drinking a cup of gynema tea an hour before eating—it supposedly makes sweet foods taste bitter, which makes it easier to pass on the chocolate dessert!

PUNCTUREVINE

• *Tribulus terristris* •

FACTS

For five thousand years, this herb has been touted as the ultimate male tonic and aphrodisiac. Today, puncturevine, also known as *tribulus*, attracts the attention of the gym crowd because it is reputed to boost testosterone levels, which can help build muscle. Some studies suggest that puncturevine can improve libido. I can't vouch for whether it does what it's supposed to do, but this herb is growing in popularity by leaps and bounds. I would caution anyone with enlarged prostate or prostate cancer to steer clear of any product that boosts testosterone, because it could worsen their condition. Buy standardized herb. Look for at least 40 percent furostanol saponin.

SHANKA PUSPI

• *Convolvulus mycrophyllus* •

FACTS

This herb is used to treat anxiety. It is also a mild painkiller.

SHATAVARI

• *Asparagus racemosus* •

FACTS

The literal translation of this herb is "[she] who possesses 100 husbands." It is the primary tonic for women and is reputed to balance female hormones at various stages of life. A secondary use is as a treatment for diabetes for both men and women.

TRIPHALA POWDER

FACTS

Triphala powder is a mixture of three dried fruits: amla, bibtaki, and haritaki. Each has been used separately or in combination to improve digestion and enhance absorption of nutrients. The most widely used preparation in Ayurvedic medicine, triphala is considered a good tonic for people of all ages. Dubbed "the good manager of the system," triphala is believed to restore balance to the body. Reputed to enhance metabolism, triphala is also touted as a weight-loss tool.

VACHA

• *Acorus calamus* •

FACTS

This herb has a calming effect on the body. It is also reputed to be an aphrodisiac.

■ Traditional Chinese Medicine

At first glance, it would appear as though traditional Chinese medicine and western herbal medicine are similar, in that they often rely on many of the same herbal remedies. There is one critical difference between the two approaches: Western herbalists, like western physicians, tend to treat ailments. They talk in concrete terms: "Have a headache? Try feverfew." Traditional Chinese healers take an entirely different approach. To them, a headache is merely a symptom of an underlying problem, which is almost always the result of a body out of balance. They would say, "Have a headache? Restore your balance and harmony, and you won't get headaches in the first place!" For centuries, each form of herbalism disdained each other's approach to healing. Recently, there have been some important changes resulting in a merger of the two traditions. For the herbal consumer, the result has been the best of both worlds.

Since the resumption of United States diplomatic relations with China in the 1970s, Westerners have been exposed to China's rich tradition of healing, which dates back more than four thousand years. Likewise, Chinese healers have learned about the spectacular medical breakthroughs in the United States that have significantly extended life. Western observers learned how traditional Chinese medicine could enhance the quality of life.

The first known Chinese medical book, the *Wu Shi Er Bing Fang, Prescriptions for Fifty-two Diseases,* was compiled around three thousand years ago. It includes 283 prescriptions for fifty-two diseases, including malaria, skin ulcers, and warts. The *Shen Nong Ben Cao Jing,* China's first bona-fide herbal, is about two thousand years old. It includes more than five hundred plants used for their medicinal purposes. The plant drugs were divided into three categories. The first group, the superior drugs, were herbs that were considered to be nontoxic and therefore were safe for daily consumption as tonics. The second group, the so-called medium drugs, were not considered entirely benign, since they could be toxic under certain circumstances. The third group, the inferior drugs, were classified as toxic, and were only used on a short-term basis to treat specific problems, much the same way we use potent antibiotics today. Many of the herbs listed in the

Shen Nong herbal are still used today in a similar fashion by Chinese physicians. The modern Chinese use some five thousand plants and animal substances as healing agents. To date, only a handful of these remedies have been seriously investigated.

The traditional Chinese approach to medicine has been not to eradicate disease, but to promote health. For example, in China, many herbs, such as ginseng, are taken as tonics: that is, they are used to enhance physical and mental well-being, not to treat a specific illness. However, in Western medicine, there are no tonics. Drugs are prescribed only for the sick, a reflection of a health-care system that is actually a sick-care system. Thanks to our exposure to traditional Chinese medicine, many western physicians are beginning to redefine their concept of the practice of medicine to include an ethic of wellness: that is, not just treating illness, but providing patients with the tools not to get sick.

Another major difference is that, in the west, medicine is considered pure science. This is not so in Asia. Chinese medicine is an interesting blend of philosophy, healing, and tradition. In western medicine, we do not recognize a drug unless it has undergone rigorous testing. The gold standard is the placebo-controlled, double-blind study. Not so in China where many of the herbs used by Chinese healers have been prescribed for hundreds, if not thousands, of years. Traditional Chinese healers recognize the validity of an herb based on a long history of use as well as anecdotal evidence. Although western scientists disdain this approach, keep in mind that our "modern medicine" is only one hundred years old; Chinese medicine is five thousand years old.

The philosophy behind traditional Chinese medicine is very complex, and it is impossible to do it justice in a few paragraphs. However, the law of yin and yang, known as "The Great Principle" to the Chinese, can shed some light on the Chinese outlook. The Chinese believe that nature is divided into two opposing cycles: yin and yang. *Yang* represents an action or activity that expends energy. *Yin* represents a more contemplative, restful phase, in which energy is replenished. The Chinese believe that maintaining a proper balance of yin and yang is essential to maintaining good health. In western terms, Chinese medicine takes a *holistic* approach to healing: Health is defined in both spiritual and physical terms.

In the west, we are just beginning to explore the relationship between body and mind and, in that respect, are light-years behind the Chinese. In recent years, we have begun to take a serious look at Chinese medicine, which may yield some promising results in terms of new drugs and therapies.

Chinese medicine focuses on using the whole herb rather than specific extracts. Very often, herbs are used in combination to treat specific problems.

The following list describes some of the most popular Chinese herbs available in the United States. Some are so popular that they are cited in the Hot Hundred. For information on how to use them, refer to the Hot Hundred listing. Although many of the better-known Chinese herbs are available at health food stores and herb shops, some of the more exotic ones are only available in Asian herb shops which, as I mentioned earlier, are generally found in urban Chinatowns. Using these herbs may require special preparation; if you want to try one of the more exotic herbs, you should consult with a Chinese herbal practitioner.

Some of the herbs listed in this section have more than one Chinese name, due to variations in dialect. Not all of the herbs are familiar to westerners or have English names.

Top Chinese Herbs

MUXU OR ZIMU

• *Western name: Alfalfa** •

FACTS

The first documented use of this herb by the Chinese dates back to the sixth century. Chinese healers use alfalfa to treat kidney stones. A mild diuretic, alfalfa is used to treat cystitis and to relieve fluid retention and swelling. (Alfalfa should not be used by people with autoimmune diseases, such as lupus or rheumatoid arthritis.)

HUANG QUI

• *Western name: Astragalus* * •

FACTS

Think of astragalus as the Chinese version of echinacea: It has been used for centuries as an immune stimulant. Only recently have western- ers begun to understand the importance of the immune system, and why herbs that keep it strong are critical to our health. Early in the twentieth century, western scientists concluded that antibiotics were the most effective way to wipe out illness. Antibiotics were distributed like candy and, as a result, we are now tackling a whole new breed of antibiotic-resistant supergerms. Thousands of years ago, Chinese heal- ers understood that the key to health was giving the body the tools it needed to fight disease on its own. They used such herbs as astragalus to strengthen the *We' Ch'i*, the body's ability to resist disease. Modern science has only recently validated their approach to preventing illness. Test tube studies have shown that astragalus can stimulate immune re- sponse against cancer cells. It makes sense that if the immune system is vigilant in weeding out troublesome cells, cancer is not allowed to take hold in the body. In animal studies, astragalus enhanced the activity of disease-fighting T-cells. When you're exposed to cold or flu germs, T-cells are the "foot soldiers" of the immune system that keep these invaders at bay. Chinese healers give astragalus to people who are run down, frequently sick, and need an immune boost.

CHUAN XIN LIAN

• *Western name: Andrographis* •

FACTS

Chinese healers have used this herb as a traditional remedy for respira- tory infections. A popular cold medicine derived from andrographis has been sold in Nordic countries for more than a decade. Andrographis is now popping up on the shelves of natural food stores in the United States as an immune stimulant and cold remedy. Researchers are investigating whether *andrographides,* compounds derived from this herb, can help treat prostate cancer. Test-tube studies have shown that these compounds can inhibit the growth of cancer cells. The next step is to test its effectiveness as a cancer fighter on animals.

BA DAN XING REN

• *Western name: Almond** •

FACTS

As far back as 200 B.C.E., the Chinese have used almond oil as a local anesthetic and muscle relaxant.

LU HUI

• *Western name: Aloe vera** •

FACTS

Aloe has been used for at least two thousand years by the Chinese. It is taken internally as a laxative, and to promote healing of disorders of the stomach, liver, and spleen. Externally, the gel is used to treat burns. Today, the Chinese use aloe gel against radiation and thermal burns, chapped and dry skin, leg ulcers, and skin disorders.

LUOLE

• *Western name: Basil** •

FACTS

Since the sixth century, basil has been used to improve blood circulation and to enhance the digestion. Externally, it is used to soothe bloodshot eyes and relieve the itching of hives.

Dou Fu

• *Western name: Tofu or bean curd* •

FACTS

Speaking of "hot," bean curd—also called *tofu*—keeps getting hotter and hotter. Tofu is a mild, white, cheeselike cake made from soymilk. Since 200 B.C.E., tofu has been cooked into a soup to treat colds—the Chinese version of chicken soup. The Japanese learned about tofu from their Chinese neighbors, and it has become a mainstay of their diet as well. Tofu is gaining in popularity in the west because it contains estrogenlike compounds called *phytoestrogens,* that may protect against many different forms of cancer. Notably, Asian women are at a significantly lower risk of dying from breast cancer than western women. Asian men are much less likely to die of prostate cancer than are western men. Many scientists believe that tofu and other soy foods are protecting Asians from cancers that are epidemic in the west.

Externally, tofu has been used to promote healing of ulcers and sores. Sold by many greengrocers, tofu is becoming popular as a meat substitute. Tofu can be stored up to five days in the refrigerator. To preserve freshness, immerse tofu in water, and change water daily. Tofu is usually added raw to hot soup, and can be sauteed in a wok with other vegetables. It is both low in calories and highly nutritious: A six-ounce portion is a mere 100 calories and contains about 6 percent protein.

YE JU

• *Western name: Chrysanthemum* •

FACTS

A homemade tea made from this flower is used to treat conjunctivitis and skin diseases. Taken internally, it is reputed to lower blood pressure. In China, dried chrysanthemum flowers are a symbol of longevity.

PU GONG YING

• *Western name: Dandelion** •

FACTS

The Chinese have known about the antibacterial properties of the juice of this flower since the seventh century. Dandelion tea is a popular treatment for upper-respiratory infections, and is sold in many health food stores and herb shops. Drink 1 cup daily.

HU SUAN

• *Western name: Garlic** •

FACTS

Garlic is popular in the United States for its cardiovascular benefits and the Chinese have used garlic as an antibiotic and an anti-inflammatory since the early sixth century. It is still an extremely popular herb in China, and is used to treat amebic dysentery, yeast infections, and middle-ear infections. Externally, it is used for nosebleeds and snake and insect bites.

GAN JIANG

• *Western name: Ginger** •

FACTS

The Chinese have used this herb to treat nausea, vomiting, and motion sickness for two thousand years. It is still one of the best remedies available for these problems. You can buy the fresh root in the produce section in most grocery stores. Commercial preparations are sold in health food stores.

REN SHEN

• *Western name: Ginseng** •

FACTS

Books have been written about this amazing herb, known as the "King of Tonics." The Chinese revere ginseng. A Chinese herbalist of 200 B.C.E. said it best, when he wrote that ginseng can "vitalize the five organs, calm the nerves, stop palpitations due to fright, brighten vision, increase intellect and with long-term use, prolong life and make one feel young."

GAN CAO

• *Western name: Licorice** •

FACTS

The Chinese have used this herb for more than five thousand years! It reduces fever and inflammation, promotes healing of wounds, and is good for sore throats and coughs. Licorice stimulates the production of bile by the liver and can relieve stomachaches and ulcers. We now know that this herb also lowers cholesterol.

FAN MU GUA

• *Western name: Papaya** •

FACTS

This herb is a sixteenth-century remedy for indigestion and constipation; it is still one of the best.

FAN JIA

• *Western name: Hot pepper (Capsicum*)* •

FACTS

An excellent source of vitamin C, the biting hot peppers typical of some Chinese cuisine have been used as a digestive aid and appetite stimulant.

MI DIE XIANG

• *Western name: Rosemary** •

FACTS

The Chinese have used this fragrant herb to treat headaches and stomachaches since the third century. It is also believed to have a calming effect on the nervous system.

BUPLERUM OR CH'AI HU

FACTS

This herb is used to bring down a fever and relieve pain. It is also believed to reduce anxiety and helps relieve nausea.

KUDZU*

• *Western name: Kudzu* •

FACTS

Chinese healers have used this herb for more than two thousand years to treat hangovers and alcoholism. Recently, researchers at Harvard Medical School have shown that kudzu can dramatically cut alcohol consumption in hamsters bred to develop an alcohol addiction similar to that of humans. Two phytochemicals in kudzu, *daidzein* and *daidzin*, help reduce blood alcohol levels. Kudzu is available in capsules.

LU RONG

• *Western name: Deer antler* •

FACTS

Since ancient times, antlers shed annually by deer have been collected by healers and used in various forms as tonics. Deer antler is reputed to contain male hormones, which could explain its reputation as an aphrodisiac. Lu rong is used in many Chinese herbal preparations, and is sold in capsule and extract form in Chinese herb shops and some health food stores. Follow package directions.

Dong Quai or Tang Kuei*
• *Western name: Chinese angelica* •

FACTS

This herb is highly valued in the Orient and, although it is called the "female ginseng," it is believed to be good for both sexes. For centuries, Chinese women have used this herb to treat gynecological problems, such as menstrual cramps and PMS. Dong quai lowers blood pressure in both men and women, and is used as a treatment for insomnia. It should never be used during pregnancy. Dong quai is available in most health food stores and herb shops in extract and capsules.

Lo Han Kuo
• *Western name: Curburbitaceae fruit* •

FACTS

Known as the "magic herb" in China, lo han kuo is a cooling herb used to balance excess yang or heat. It is a traditional treatment for sore throats, hacking coughs, and poor digestion. Today, it is included in many herbal Chinese formulas, and is available as a tea.

Cordonopsis
• *Western name: Cordonopsis tangshen* •

FACTS

This herb is considered a milder version of ginseng and is used as a tonic and an energizer. It is used as a substitute for ginseng, especially for those who find ginseng to be too strong. Cordonopsis is also good for digestion and heartburn. This herb is sold as a tea or in capsules.

ZHI SHI

• *Western name: Immature bitter orange*
(Citrus aurantium) •

FACTS

Zhi shi has been used for thousands of years by Chinese healers to treat allergies, digestive problems, and colds. *Syneprine,* its active ingredient, is a weaker relative of ephedra. Similar to ephedra, it is being used in weight-loss products to increase metabolic rate. Since it is not as strong as ephedra, it is reputed to have fewer untoward side effects. Keep in mind, however, that it is still a mild stimulant, and may make some people jumpy. (See *Ma huang.*)

MA HUANG

• *Western name: Ephedra** •

FACTS

The Chinese have traditionally used this herb to treat asthma. Today, compounds derived from this herb are commonly found in many over-the-counter cold and allergy medications. Ephedra is also a long-acting stimulant, and should not be used by people with high blood pressure. American ephedra, known as *Mormon* tea or *desert* tea, is much milder than the Chinese variety and is used in a similar fashion. Ma huang is used in many natural cold remedies.

HO SHOU WU FO-TI

FACTS

Ho shou wu is known in China as a longevity herb. The Chinese believe that it is a rejuvenating tonic that can help preserve youthful vigor and energy. It is also believed to prevent gray hair and promote fertility in both sexes. Chinese studies show that extracts of this herb have anti-tumor properties. Ho shou wu is believed to prevent blood clots, lower blood pressure, and strengthen the heart. This herb is widely available in capsule and extract form in health food stores and herb shops.

DA T'SAO
• *Western name: Jujube date* •

FACTS

This herb has a calming effect on the body, and is used to treat insomnia and dizziness. Jujube is sold in Chinese herb shops.

KOU CHI TZA
• *Western name: Lycii* •

FACTS

This herb is believed to increase longevity and promote cheerfulness. Chinese physicians use it as a treatment for high blood pressure, kidney disease, and some forms of cancer. Lycii can be found in most Chinese herb shops.

Pai Shu

FACTS

This herb is known for its diuretic properties and can be found in many Chinese herb shops.

Jie Eng

• *Western name: Platycodon* •

FACTS

This herb is used to treat respiratory problems such as asthma, coughs, and bronchitis. It is also used for sore throats and lung ailments. Platycodon can be found at most Chinese herb shops.

Ko Ken

• *Western name: Pueraria* •

FACTS

Chinese healers use this herb to treat colds, flu, and gastrointestinal problems. It can be purchased in Chinatowns or in natural food stores.

Rehmannia E

FACTS

This herb is used to treat anemia, fatigue, and to promote the healing of injured bones. It is sold in Chinese herb shops.

DANG SHEN

• *Western name: Salvia* •

FACTS

Chinese women use this herb to promote menstrual regularity. It is sold in Chinese herb shops.

SCHIZANDRA FRUCTUS OR SCHIZANDRA CHINENSIS

FACTS

This herb is highly prized by Chinese women as a sexual enhancer and youth tonic. It is believed to preserve beauty and is a mild sedative. Schizandra is also reputed to increase sexual stamina among men. Until recently, this herb was rare and relatively expensive. It was highly coveted by the wealthy and was a favorite among the Chinese emperors. Schizandra is also considered an adaptogen and, similar to ginseng, it is believed to increase stamina and fight fatigue. It is also being touted as an antidepressant. Recent research supports some of these claims. According to a 1989 article in *Phytotherapy Research,* polo ponies given schizandra performed better and showed better physiological responses to stress after taking the herb. Today, schizandra is widely available at health food stores and herb shops in capsules and extract. Follow package directions.

FANG-FENG
....
• *Western name: Sileris* •

FACTS

This herb is used to treat muscle spasms, and is reputed to bolster the immune system. It can be found at most Chinese herb shops.

■ South American Herbs

Ever since the first European explorers set foot in the New World, South America has been a fertile ground for plant medicines. To this day, much of the South American population still relies on herbal remedies. In urban centers in the United States with large Hispanic communities, the neighborhood botanica or herb shop often does a brisker business than the local pharmacy. Many herbs commonly used in the United States originated in South America; however, there are scores of others that have not yet found their way here. The following is a list of the hottest South American herbs. Some are already household names; the others, I predict, are destined to become so. Although this list includes some Hot Hundred herbs that are widely available in packaged form, some of the more obscure herbs may be sold in their natural state and require preparation. Be sure to check with a knowledgeable herbal practitioner before using an unfamiliar herb.

CAJUEIRO

FACTS

Rich in vitamin C, cajueiro, also known as *cashew fruit,* is an old time remedy for colds and flus. It is now popping up in herbal formulas designed to boost energy and sexual function.

CAYENNE*
• *Capsicum anuun, Capsicum frutescens* •

FACTS

Native to northeastern coastal areas of South America, these red-hot peppers have been used in folk medicine since 7000 B.C.E.! Studies show that hot peppers are heart healthy. They can trim cholesterol and triglyceride levels. Used externally in a cream or ointment, they can help reduce the pain of post shingles and arthritis. A spicy meal is a great way to clear a stuffy nose!

GUARANA*
• *Paulina cupana* •

FACTS

The seeds of this plant contain up to 5 percent caffeine and are well known for their stimulating effect. Guarana is reputed to increase mental alertness and fight fatigue. In Brazil, guarana is used in soft drinks. It is available in the United States in capsule form, by itself, or in combination with other herbs. Follow package directions or consult an herbal practitioner.

IPECAC
• *Cephaelis ipecacuanha* •

FACTS

Found in southwestern Brazil, this herb induces vomiting and, there-fore, is a popular remedy for food poisoning and other kinds of poisoning. Syrup of ipecac is approved by the FDA and is sold in drugstores. The herb itself is very toxic except when diluted in syrup form. Because it induces vomiting, ipecac is often abused by teenage girls suffering from *bulimia,* an eating disorder characterized by gorging and purging. Although this herb is an essential for every household, doctors recommend that you do not keep it accessible to teenagers who may be tempted to use it to lose weight.

> **CAUTION** It is not always appropriate to induce vomiting in cases of poisoning. Check with your physician or local poison-alert hotline before giving this or any other drug to a poison victim.

MATE
• *Ilex paraguarienesis* •

FACTS

Once used as a folk remedy against scurvy, a beverage made out of the leaf of this plant is the national drink of Argentina. Mate contains caffeine as well as vitamins C, A, and B complex. In Argentina, mate is touted as an energizer and a tonic. In fact, it is so popular that the average Argentinian consumes about eleven pounds of mate annually.

MUIRA PUAMA
• *Ptychopetalum olacoides* •

FACTS

The bark and roots of this plant are highly regarded by the Brazilians as a stimulant, stomach tonic, and treatment for rheumatism. This herb is reputed to be an aphrodisiac. Although muira puama is very popular in Brazil, it is just being discovered in the United States.

Pau D'Arco*
• *Tabecuia impetiginosa* •

FACTS

Also known as *taheebo, lapacho,* and *ipe roxo,* this herb is a folk remedy in Brazil for cancer and fungal infections. Studies show that this herb indeed has antitumor and antifungal properties. Pau d'arco is widely available in the United States in capsules and extract form.

Sarsaparilla*
• *Smilax officinalis* •

FACTS

Native to Central America, this herb was a popular flavor in root beers and soft drinks at the turn of the century. It is currently used in the United States by bodybuilders as a nonsteroidal method of increasing muscle mass, and is also touted as an aphrodisiac. However, chemical analysis has not found any evidence of testosterone or other male hormones in this herb.

Stevia
• *Stevia rebaudiana* •

FACTS

Originally from Paraguay, this herb is two hundred times sweeter than sugar. It is used in Japan as a noncaloric sweetener, but has not been approved for this use in the United States. Dried stevia leaves and liquid preparations are available at botanicas and health food stores.

SUMA*
• *Pfaffia paniculata* •

F A C T S

This herb is an extremely popular tonic in Brazil, and is also used by women there to relieve the symptoms associated with menopause. As the baby-boom generation reaches menopause within the next decade, I predict that this herb, along with others that are reputed to ease the transition to menopause, will increase in popularity in the United States.

WILD MEXICAN YAM
• *Diosorea mexicanan* and *Diosorea composita* •

F A C T S

Used by native Mexican women for birth control and to prevent miscarriage, this yam produces chemicals from which oral contraceptives and sex hormones are synthesized. Some women herbalists in the United States use an extract from this herb as a contraceptive. I do not advise using this or any other herb to prevent conception, unless under the supervision of a qualified practitioner.

NATIVE AMERICAN HERBS

If there were no plants, we wouldn't be here. We breathe in what they breathe out. That is how we learn from them.

—K E E T W U A H, *a well-known Cherokee healer*

When early settlers arrived in the United States there were more than two thousand tribes of Native Americans. Each tribe had its own system of herbal medicine that was, in many ways, far superior to the European style of health care practiced by the pioneers. In fact, early settlers were startled to see Indians recovering from injuries that they considered to be fatal. Noted one observer, "I have seen many who have received four or five bullet or arrow wounds through the stomach and who are so perfectly cured of them that they do not suffer any inconvenience. Through the knowledge of simples [herbs] which they received from their fathers, they will cure hands, arms, and feet that our best surgeons would not hesitate to cut."

The typical tribal medicine man was as well equipped as any modern pharmacy to treat a wide range of medical needs, ranging from the common cold to birth control. Although we have incorporated some Native American herbs into our herbal tradition—in fact, some have even made it into the Hot Hundred—many have been forgotten or are difficult to obtain. Although you will not be able to locate most of these herbs at the local health food store, I have included a list of Native American herbal remedies for common problems to show how sophisticated this culture really was.

Colds

Wungobe	Balsam fir
Nakadonup	Wild buckwheat

Ya-Tombe	Creosote bush
Aqui he binga	Blue gilia
Toza	Indian balsam
Taba emul	Meadow rye
Toya bawana	Horsemint
Batipi	Wild peony

Sore Throat

Ax six sixie	Bitterroot
Pakitoki	Double bladder pod
Quit chemboo	Licorice root*
Pooy sonib	String plant
A sat chiot sake	Rattle weed

Eye Problems

Apos-ipoco	Alum root
So yaits	Pink plumes
Pah oh pimb	Acacia or cat claw
Sebu mogoonobu	Back turtle

Kidney and Bladder Ailments

Poku erop	Iris flag
Kube	Sage, bud
Sammapo	Juniper berry*

Laxatives

Bossowey	Sweet anise*
Ae buchoko	Cascara sagrada*
Kosi tube	Gray willow

Rheumatism

Wapi	Juniper berry*
Pennikinni	Wormwood
Yano	Wild rose

Toothache

Poku erop	Iris
Pannonzia	Yarrow
Segumogoonbu	Nettleback

Chewing Gum

Wahanane	Desert gum plant

Shampoo

Datil or viemp	Yucca*
Amole Indian	Soap root

An Old Remedy for an Old Problem

In 1983, public-health officials in Beijing, China, announced that a four-hundred-year-old prescription for treating hemorrhoids had been tested on forty thousand patients and proved to be 96 percent effective. The remedy: the injection of insect secretions on sumac leaves combined with crystal salts.

SAVING A TREASURE

Since the *Herb Bible* was published in 1992, the world's rain forests have been vanishing. Within the past few decades, we have witnessed the destruction of half of the world's tropical rain forests. Every second, another 1.5 acres of rainforest disappears—adding up to fifty million acres per year. Deforestation is occurring at an alarming rate to make way for farming, logging, and other industries. This is very short-sighted, considering that these natural areas are potential treasure troves of new pharmaceuticals. Every acre that is burned to create lumber or condominiums represents the loss of a potential cure. Could we already have rid the world of the cure for cancer? Is there a treatment for AIDS hidden deep within the forest? We may never know. If present trends continue, by the first quarter of the twenty-first century, the tropical rain forest will become as extinct as the dinosaur. As more and more of this precious land is plundered by developers for its minerals and lumber, countless species of plants and animals are also doomed to extinction.

Unfortunately, we are decimating the plant life faster than we can study it. Less than 1 percent of all tropical rain-forest plants have been adequately researched for their medicinal properties. This is especially tragic in light of the fact that 25 percent of all Western medicines are derived from rain-forest plants. A whopping 70 percent of the three thousand plant species known for their anticancer properties originated in the rainforest. Tropical plants such as the rosy periwinkle have given us two of our most powerful weapons against cancer—vincristine and vinblastine. The pilocarpus tree, native to South America, spawned a highly effective treatment for glaucoma.

Many of these "wonder drugs" were brought to our attention by the local medicine men or shamans, the main health-care providers in these remote areas. As the rainforests are flattened by bulldozers, the secrets of the shamans will be lost forever, along with numerous plant cures that could have saved countless lives.

CHAPTER 5

The Herbal
Medicine Cabinet

Centuries *before our* medicine cabinets were jammed with
over-the-counter medicines, our ancestors were treating themselves
and their families with healing agents derived from the plant kingdom.
There was an herbal remedy for just about every malady known to
man, woman, and child—from fever to fatigue—and many worked
surprisingly well. In this chapter, I have compiled a list of some home
remedies that I feel still belong in the modern medicine cabinet.

When is it appropriate to self-medicate with an herb, and when
should you seek medical advice? Whether you are using standard over-
the-counter medications or herbal therapies, the same common-sense
rules apply. If you have a cold, flu, headache, or minor scrape or bug
bite, you probably don't have to call your physician. If a problem
persists, however, or if a new problem develops, you should seek medical advice. Obviously, if you have a persistent fever or cough, unusual
headache, or experience untoward symptoms such as dizziness, loss of
vision, fainting, chest pain or anything out of the ordinary, call for help.

Since the publication of the first edition of the *Herb Bible,* there
have been many more herbal combination products brought to market
designed to treat specific ailments, such as colds, arthritis symptoms,
allergies, mild depression, and headaches. Many of these products are
quite effective, but be sure to read the label carefully so you know all the
ingredients. You don't want to take an herb that you may be allergic to,
or is contraindicated for other reasons. (Do not give any herbs to children without first consulting with your pediatrician. Herbs listed in the

Hot Hundred are designated by an asterisk. See the Hot Hundred entries for more information.)

The Best Herbs for Colds, Coughs, and Flus

Most people will get from three to six colds a year, and countless others
will be stricken with flu. Given the fact that hundreds of different
viruses can cause a cold, and that new flu strains crop up each year, the
odds of defeating these viral pests are slim. Sure, we can keep ourselves
strong so that we are not susceptible to every cough and cold that
comes our way. If we do get sick, however, we need to know how to relieve our symptoms and regain our health as quickly as possible. Here
are my favorite remedies for those troublesome bugs.

HOT TEA AND HONEY.   Drink several cups of your favorite decaffeinated tea. Add a tablespoon of honey. It will not only soothe your
throat, but is loaded with immune-stimulating antioxidants. (For extra
vitamin C, drink rose-hip tea. Marshmallow-root and raspberry-leaf
tea are especially kind to a sore throat.)

ELDERBERRY.*   Studies suggest that elderberry syrup and lozenges can
reduce the severity of respiratory symptoms and duration of viral infections. Take 1 tablespoon of elderberry extract, or one lozenge every
four hours for up to four days. (It is also available in capsule form.)

ECHINACEA,* AMERICAN FEVERFEW,* AND GOLDENSEAL.*   Fight
back! Echinacea will give your immune system a much-needed boost.
Goldenseal has mild antibiotic activity, and helps clear congestion due
to inflammation of the mucus membranes. Feverfew can bring down a
fever. Look for herbal combination formulas containing these three
herbs. Do not take for more than two weeks at a time.

OLIVE LEAF EXTRACT.*   Olive leaf extract contains *elenolic acid,* a natural antibacterial/antiviral compound. For colds and flu, take three 500
mg. capsules every four hours.

EUCALYPTUS.   Use 1 to 5 drops of eucalyptus oil in a vaporizer to produce a soothing steam that helps clear clogged nasal passages.

FENUGREEK TEA.*   This tea is a good expectorant and is also soothing for sore throats. Fenugreek is available in dried herb, extract, and in tea bags. For tea, use 1 teaspoon dried herb in hot water. Use 10 to 20 drops of the extract in warm water. Add 1 teaspoon of honey for a soothing drink.

MULLEIN TEA.   Try a cup for dry, nagging coughs. Use 1 tablespoon of the dried herb in 1 cup hot water. Drink up to 2 cups of this tea daily to relieve symptoms.

BEE PROPOLIS.*   Empty two bee-propolis capsules in warm water. Mix until dissolved. Use as a gargle to relieve throat pain. It is also a natural antiseptic.

SLIPPERY ELM BARK.*   These lozenges help relieve sore-throat pain.

■ Herbs to Bring Down a Fever

A fever is a sign that the immune system has been activated, and that the body is trying to "cook" an infection. There are two schools of thought about bringing down a fever. Some old-time herbalists feel that a low-grade fever should be allowed to run its course. Others feel that view is archaic, subjecting the patient to needless suffering. Here's my position. First, if you have a high fever (over 102) for more than 24 hours, call your physician for advice. Unless you have other symptoms or a pre-existing condition, your doctor will probably tell you to try the standard home remedies before coming to see him or her. Nevertheless, you should call. Second, if you have a low-grade fever and are not uncomfortable, simply sleep it off. Very often, bed rest and hot drinks will help you recover. If you are uncomfortable, however, by all means try these simple steps to bring the fever down.

WHITE WILLOW BARK.*   This precursor to modern-day aspirin helps break a fever. Take 2 capsules every 3 hours as needed.

FEVERFEW.*   As its name implies, another old-time remedy to bring down a fever. Take 1 to 3 capsules until temperature is normal.

BARBERRY.   A cup of barberry tea promotes sweating and helps to cool the body. Mix 3 to 7 drops of extract in ¹/₂ cup water. Drink up to 3 times daily.

▪ Herbs for Allergies

About 35 million Americans suffer from some form of allergy. Hay fever and other seasonal allergies are the most common, and there are numerous over the counter remedies. Unfortunately, many can cause unpleasant side effects such as jitteriness, dry mouth, and/or drowsiness. Try these herbal remedies: There are no known side effects and, if they work for you, they can spare you from having to take anything stronger.

STINGING NETTLE.*   There is much anecdotal evidence that this herb can relieve allergic symptoms, such as teary eyes and runny nose. Take 1 to 2 capsules or tablets, up to 4 times daily as needed. Do not take nettle if you have untreated high blood pressure.

BROMELAIN* AND QUERCETIN.   *Bromelain is* an enzyme found in pineapple that is a natural anti-inflammatory. *Quercetin* is a bioflavonoid found in onion and garlic that can help stop the allergic pathway in the body. Together, they spell relief for many allergy sufferers. Take separately, or try a combination formula.

EYEBRIGHT.*   An eyewash made from this herb is good for allergic, itchy eyes. Mix 1 tablespoon herb in 1 cup hot water. Let cool. Use on eyes as needed.

Herbs for Good Digestion

If you find yourself popping antacids before or after every meal, here are some natural solutions.

PAPAYA.*   Papaya tablets can help relieve indigestion. Take 1 tablet up to 3 times daily. Or eat some fresh papaya slices. They're delicious!

BROMELAIN.*   A protein-digesting enzyme group found in pineapple, bromelain helps the absorption of nutrients. Take 1 to 2 tablets after meals.

BASIL.*   This herb is good for a gassy stomach. Mix 1 teaspoon of dried herb in $^1/_2$ cup warm water. Strain. Drink 1 to 2 cups daily.

CARAWAY.   This is a time-tested remedy for indigestion. Mix 3 to 4 drops of extract in 1 cup liquid. Drink 3 to 4 times daily as needed.

CHAMOMILE.*   A cup of chamomile tea is good for indigestion and has a calming effect on the body. Drink 1 cup nightly.

DILL.   This herb is excellent for gas and indigestion. Steep 2 teaspoons of dill seeds in 1 cup warm water for 10 to 15 minutes. Strain. Drink $^1/_2$ cup up to 3 times daily.

FENNEL.*   Fennel tea can relieve gas and cramps. Mix 10 to 20 drops of extract in 1 cup warm water. Sweeten with honey. Drink 2 to 3 cups, as needed.

Herbal Remedies for Nausea and Vomiting

Everyone has experienced that nauseated, sick feeling at one time or another. When it strikes, here are some ways to make yourself feel better.

GINGER TEA.* Ginger is a proven antinauseant. For many people, a cup or two of ginger tea is all it takes. It is particularly good for morning sickness.

PEPPERMINT TEA.* A cup of peppermint tea will quell stomach cramps and nausea.

CINNAMON. Cinnamon is excellent for upset stomach, gas, and diarrhea. Put a few drops of cinnamon oil in warm water. Drink as needed.

Herbs for Constipation

First and foremost, if you eat a diet high in fiber, you can avoid becoming constipated in the first place. Unfortunately, the typical American diet is filled with refined, overly processed foods, devoid of nutrients and fiber. Although I trust that most of the readers of this book are health conscious enough to eat sensibly, there are undoubtedly times when you can't. Stress, illness, or even certain medications can cause constipation. Drink eight glasses of water daily—it can help keep you regular. Avoid synthetic laxatives, as they can cause dependency. In addition, try these herbal solutions.

CASCARA. For occasional problems, this herb is an excellent laxative. Cascara is available in capsule form. Do not exceed recommended dose. It is not for everyday use.

PSYLLIUM.* Adding psyllium to your diet will help keep you regular. Put 1 teaspoon in 1 cup water or juice, and drink 2 to 3 cups daily, or take psyllium capsules. Drink at least 8 glasses of water throughout the day.

▪ Herbs to Stop Diarrhea and Cramping

Mild diarrhea and cramping can be treated with the following herbs:

APPLE.*   A grated, peeled apple* is good for diarrhea.

CATNIP.   Not just for cats! Catnip tea can help relieve diarrhea. Mix 1 tablespoon dried herb in 8 ounces hot water.

ARROWROOT.   Arrowroot is good for an upset stomach. Mix 2 teaspoons in 2 cups warm water. Flavor with honey or cinnamon. Drink 2 cups daily.

CARROTS.*   Eating 3 grated, raw carrots works well for diarrhea. The pectin will help slow down the GI tract.

▪ Herbal Diuretics

Bloating or fluid retention should always be checked by a physician, because it could be a sign of a more serious problem. However, in many cases, it is not and can be handled quite effectively with dietary changes (cut down on the salt!) and the right herbs. In particular, women may notice that they retain fluid right before their periods. This is due to hormonal changes that can be modulated by herbs. Beware of synthetic diuretics: They can be harsh to the system and can destroy the normal mineral balance in the body.

ALFALFA.   Alfalfa (tea or tablets) is a mild diuretic. It is safe for just about everyone, with the exception of people with autoimmune problems such as lupus or rheumatoid arthritis.

DANDELION.*   This herb is a natural diuretic that is also rich in potassium. Drink a cup of dandelion tea, eat fresh greens, or take up to 3 capsules daily as needed.

JUNIPER BERRY.   Juniper berry is an excellent diuretic. Mix 10 to 20 drops of extract in 1 cup liquid. Take 2 to 3 times as needed.

Herbs for Toothache

Have a toothache? Call your dentist! Here's what you can do before you see him or her to make yourself more comfortable.

CLOVES.   Put 2 to 5 drops of clove oil on affected area.

Herbal Mouthwashes

If you have a breath problem, try these mouthwashes. Do not suck on mints or other sweet candies during the day—they will damage your teeth and gums.

BARBERRY.   This herb strengthens weak gums. Mix 3 to 7 drops of extract in 1/2 cup water. Rinse 3 times daily.

GOLDENSEAL.*   A mouthwash made out of goldenseal powder and water is excellent for sore gums and helps prevent gum disease.

NEEM.*   This Ayurvedic herb is used to strengthen gums, prevent tooth decay, and fight the bacteria that cause bad breath. Look for neem mouthwash.

GREEN TEA.*   Green tea contains compounds that kill the bacteria that cause both bad breath and tooth decay. Sip a cup of tea after your meal.

MYRRH.   Since biblical times, myrrh has been used for irritated and infected gums and canker sores. Mix 2 to 5 drops in 1 cup water. Use as needed.

■ Herbal Moisturizers

Dry, itchy skin is a very common problem, especially in the winter, when it can be aggravated by the combination of cold air and hot, dry heat. As we age, levels of important hormones decline, which can also dry out skin. Very often, harsh soaps and cleansers can aggravate the problem. Use only gentle cleansers: Chamomile cleansers work well without stripping your skin of its natural oils. Be sure to moisturize your skin from within by drinking 8 glasses of water daily. Also, follow these other helpful tips:

FLAXSEED OIL.   Flaxseed oil is a rich source of omega 3 fatty acids, which can help keep your skin from drying out. Take 2 tablespoons of flaxseed oil daily, or the equivalent in flaxseed oil capsules. Store in re-frigerator.

ALOE GEL.*   Pure aloe gel is great first aid for rough, dry skin.

ALMOND OIL.*   Is great for rough spots, such as the soles of your feet!

■ Herbs for Sunburn

Gently rub any of these herbs on the burned area.

GREEN TEA.*   Make a cup of green tea and let it cool. Dab the cool tea on the sunburned area. It will not only soothe the sore, burning sensa-tion, but the antioxidants in the tea will help repair the damaged skin.

ALOE GEL.*   This herb will cool and soothe. Apply to skin 3 times daily, as needed.

WITCH HAZEL.   Dab a little witch hazel on the affected area 3 times daily, as needed.

Herbs for Minor Burns

You accidentally burn your hand on a hot pot, or scald your hand in hot water. It may not be serious enough to call your doctor, but it sure hurts! First, run cold water over the affected area to relieve the burn. Then, try these herbal remedies.

ALOE GEL.*   This herb relieves pain and promotes healing of burns.

HONEY.   The kind you put in tea is terrific for minor burns. The antioxidants in honey promote fast healing.

GINGER ROOT.*   The juice from crushed ginger root relieves that hot, stinging sensation.

Herbs for Skin Irritations

Keep these herbs in stock for scrapes, bruises, and other minor skin irritations.

ARNICA.*   Arnica lotion promotes healing of wounds. Use daily, only on unbroken skin!

CALENDULA.   Derived from marigold, this salve and ointment is soothing to skin wounds and bruises. Follow package directions.

ECHINACEA OIL.*   This natural disinfectant can be applied directly to minor cuts and wounds.

COMFREY.*   This salve or ointment promotes healing of scrapes, cuts, and other skin wounds. Follow package directions.

ALOE GEL.*   This herb is good for almost any kind of minor skin wound. Use as needed.

■ Herbs for Arthritis and Muscle Aches

You wake up sore and stiff. Maybe you have arthritis, or maybe you worked out too much the day before. Here are some herbal solutions to this very common problem. Herbs taken by mouth may not work as fast as over-the-counter pain relievers, but they are far gentler. Herbal preparations applied directly to the sore muscle or joint are quite effective, but not long-lasting.

BOSWELLIA.*   An ointment made from this Ayurvedic herb can be rubbed directly into the sore muscle or joint. Taken orally, over time, boswellia may help relieve some of the symptoms of arthritis.

EUCALYPTUS.   Liniments made from this herb are very soothing to sore, inflamed joints. Apply to affected area.

CAPSAICIN CREAM.*   For fast relief, try a cream made from the active ingredient of cayenne pepper. Some people with very sensitive skin may find capsaicin cream to be irritating.

GINGER COMBINATION.*   I take an herbal extract of several subspecies of the ginger plant for maximum relief. It will work in 3 to 5 days.

EVENING PRIMROSE OIL.*   Take 2 to 3 capsules evening primrose oil daily to relieve arthritis pain.

TURMERIC.*   A main ingredient of curry, turmeric is a well-known anti-inflammatory that has been used for arthritis. Take 1 (300 mg.) capsule up to 3 times daily.

WHITE WILLOW BARK.*   An anti-inflammatory, white willow bark is used to relieve muscle aches and sprains, as well as arthritis. Take 2 capsules every 3 hours, as needed.

BROMELAIN.* Derived from fresh pineapple, bromelain is a natural anti-inflammatory that can help relieve the aches and pains of arthritis. Take 2 (500 mg.) capsules daily.

Herbal Headache Remedies

After the common cold, headache is probably the most common complaint typically treated with over-the-counter remedies.

FEVERFEW.* This herb not only helps to prevent migraine headaches, but can stop a headache before it hits. If you feel a headache coming on, take 2 capsules and lay down.

WHITE WILLOW BARK.* This herb is an excellent aspirin substitute. Available in tablet form, take 2 capsules every 3 hours, as needed.

PEPPERMINT TEA.* A cup of peppermint tea is soothing for a headache, and that nauseated feeling that may accompany it.

Herbs for Dizziness and Motion Sickness

A sudden bout of dizziness should be reported to your physician. However, many people suffer from periodic episodes of vertigo and motion sickness, for which there are few effective treatments. These herbs may help relieve the unpleasant symptoms.

GINKGO BILOBA.* This ancient herb is excellent for chronic dizziness and lightheadedness. Take 3 capsules daily.

GINGER.* Ginger tea, tablets, or capsules are terrific for motion sickness. Take 1 standardized extract capsule up to 3 times daily.

Herbs for Earaches

Severe earaches, especially those in children, should be treated by a physician. Mild earaches can be dealt with effectively at home.

GARLIC OIL.* A few drops of garlic oil from a garlic capsule (a combination of garlic oil and other vegetable oils) can help an earache. Undiluted garlic oil is too strong.

ECHINACEA* AND AMERICAN FEVERFEW.* These immune-boosting herbs can help the body fight the infection causing the earache. Take 5 tablets daily for 5 to 7 days.

CALENDULA EARDROPS. An oil made of calendula can help soothe the pain.

Herbal Breath Fresheners

Try these natural ways to keep your breath fresh.

GREEN TEA.* Sip a cup of green tea after meals when you can't brush your teeth. It will help kill bacteria that promotes bad breath, cavities, and gum disease.

PARSLEY.* Often used as a garnish, a parsley sprig is a terrific breath freshener.

Herbal Deodorants

Try eliminating body odor from the inside out!

CHLORELLA TABLETS. Chlorella tablets can help eliminate body odor. Take 1 to 3 tablets daily.

Herbs for Skin Rashes

Some people have never had a skin rash in their lives, and others are constantly plagued by them. There are numerous treatments for skin rashes, but many contain steroids, anti-inflammatory compounds that, over time, can thin the skin. These herbal skin remedies may work just as well for you, but without the troublesome side effects.

OREGON GRAPE. This herb is a traditional treatment for skin inflammations, including psoriasis. In Germany, an external ointment from this herb has yielded good results. Try it, and see if it works for you.

BLACK WALNUT. An extract of this herb is an old-time remedy for psoriasis. Try rubbing the extract directly on affected areas twice a day.

GOLDENSEAL.* This herb is a folk cure for eczema. Rub extract on dry, red patches daily.

EVENING PRIMROSE OIL.* This natural anti-inflammatory is recommended for psoriasis, eczema, and other skin conditions.

Herbs That Promote Sleep

Of all the things you can do to preserve your health, getting a good night's sleep tops the list. Sleep not only leaves you feeling energized and recharged, but helps build your resistance to disease by bolstering your immune system. Try these herbal remedies to help you sleep better.

CHAMOMILE TEA.* A cup of chamomile tea is very relaxing at night.

VALERIAN.* This herb is particularly good for nervous insomnia and anxiety. Take 2 capsules before bedtime, or drink a cup of valerian tea.

PASSION FLOWER.*   Often used in combination with valerian, passion flower can help lull you to sleep. Drink a cup of tea, or take 2 capsules before bedtime.

■ Herbal Stress Busters

As a pharmacist, I know that synthetic tranquilizers work, but are often accompanied by some unpleasant side effects, ranging from dry mouth to nausea. For many people, an herb may do the job without any side effects. These are the herbs I believe are best for reducing stress.

KAVA.*   This herb from the South Pacific can reduce anxiety and lull you into a good mood. Use it only at night, before bed time. Take 1 to 2 capsules before bedtime.

HOPS.   This is an old favorite. Mix ½ teaspoon dried herb in ½ cup water. Drink daily. Sprinkle dry hops on your pillow.

PASSION FLOWER.*   This herb is especially good for times of acute anxiety. Mix 15 to 60 drops of extract in liquid. Drink daily. Do not use during pregnancy.

VALERIAN.*   Nature's own tranquilizer! Take 1 to 3 capsules daily, or 10 drops extract in liquid.

SKULLCAP.*   This herb is one of the oldest remedies for stress. Use 1 teaspoon of dried herb in 1 cup hot water for a home-brewed tea. Mix 3 to 12 drops extract in liquid daily. Take 1 capsule up to 3 times daily.

ST. JOHN'S WORT.*   I recommend this herb in combination with a polyphenol complex for acute stress. It works fast!

■ Herbal Energizers

Get a natural lift from these herbs!

CAYENNE.* This herb has a mild stimulating effect. Try a cup of cayenne tea when you're feeling tired and run down.

GINSENG.* If used consistently, ginseng (panax, American, or Siberian) can help eliminate fatigue. Ginseng is available in capsules, extract, or tea.

■ Herbs for Athlete's Foot

This is one of the most annoying problems known to man (and woman)! Try these herbal remedies.

TEA TREE.* The ointment or oil, which is sold in most health food stores, is a traditional remedy for this fungal infection. Follow package directions. Keep your feet dry by changing your shoes and socks several times daily.

APPLE CIDER VINEGAR. An old folk remedy for athlete's foot. Rub on affected areas several times a day. It might sting a little at first, but persevere; it is effective.

OREGANO OIL.* Try this natural antifungal for athlete's foot. Apply directly to affected area. Use daily.

Jewish Penicillin? It Can't Hurt

In the twelfth century, the great physician and philosopher, Maimonides, prescribed herbal baths and chicken soup as remedies for the common cold. Mothers have been following his advice ever since—at least the chicken soup part. More than eight hundred years later, the *New England Journal of Medicine* confirmed that Maimonides was right. Researchers found that chicken soup was a mild antibiotic and decongestant. Chinese healers also use chicken soup to treat colds, but they add a little ginseng to their brew. Throw in some shiitake mushrooms for a delicious immune boost.

Look for a new product in the natural food stores—herbal chicken soup. It contains echinacea, astragalus, and vitamin C in the soup. What, no antioxidant-enriched matzoh balls?

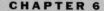

CHAPTER 6

A Woman's Body

Modern medicine has been a predominantly male profession. In fact, it was only within the past few decades that medical schools began admitting women in equal numbers with men. Ironically, however, the first healers were probably women, and the drugs they used were the seeds, leaves, berries, and bark they collected for food. It's not surprising that women would have taken such an active interest in healing. Their unique biology and hormonal cycles made it all the more important for them to have a basic understanding of herbal medicine. Unfortunately, much of this knowledge has been lost and the rich tradition of the wise-woman healer is fast becoming a thing of the past. Women constantly ask me about natural alternatives to the drugs and procedures that are typically used for women's problems. Here are some of the questions that women commonly ask me about herbs.

▓ Menopause

Since I've recently become menopausal, I have suffered from symptoms such as frequent hot flashes, insomnia, and joint pain. My doctor prescribed hormone-replacement therapy, but I am reluctant to take hormones because I am worried about breast cancer. I am also concerned about osteoporosis, which can be helped by taking hormones. Are there any herbs that I can try instead?

This is probably the number one question that I am asked by women of all ages. On the one hand, hormone-replacement therapy can not only reduce the discomfort of menopause, but protects against bone loss associated with osteoporosis. On the other hand, several studies have found that taking hormones may increase the risk of developing breast cancer. The decision whether to take hormones should be made by the woman and a knowledgeable physician or natural healer who can review her options. Here are some things to consider.

The sudden drop in estrogen levels is responsible for many of the annoying symptoms that women experience during menopause, including hot flashes, mood swings, and headaches. Most of these symptoms disappear on their own within a year or two but, for some women, it can be a year or two of pure torture. Many women find that hormone-replacement therapy—supplemental estrogen and progesterone—makes them feel like themselves again. There are, however, several problems with hormone replacement. First, some women experience unpleasant side effects similar to PMS, such as bloating and headaches. Second, as I mentioned earlier, estrogen replacement has been linked to an added risk of breast cancer in some studies. Fortunately, there are several herbs that can help ease menopausal symptoms without side effects or the added cancer risk. Black cohosh has become the herb of choice for treating common menopausal symptoms. This herb works by inhibiting the production of luteinizing hormone (LH), the cause of much menopausal discomfort. Several European studies document that black cohosh can work as well, if not better, than standard hormone-replacement therapy. The usual dose is 40 mg. black cohosh daily; most women feel better within 2 to 3 weeks. Since we don't know the long term effects of black cohosh, I don't recommend taking it for more than six months; however, by that time, your symptoms may disappear on their own. Black cohosh should also help relieve menopausal insomnia but, if it doesn't, try taking two valerian capsules at night. In addition, take 400 IU of natural vitamin E (in the form of mixed tocopherol) daily to help control hot flashes.

Many women find that ginseng can also greatly relieve the hot flashes and other unpleasant side effects associated with menopause. Try 1 capsule up to 3 times daily or 1 cup ginseng tea every day. In rare cases, ginseng may stimulate vaginal bleeding which, in this case, is harmless but can be quite frightening. Any kind of vaginal bleeding after menstruation may be a warning sign of cancer and should be reported immediately to your physician. However, make sure that your physician knows that you've been using ginseng.

About one in four women will develop osteoporosis after menopause. *Osteoporosis* is characterized by the thinning of bone, which leaves it more vulnerable to fractures. To preserve your bone, be sure to get enough bone-building calcium and magnesium in your diet and in supplements. Yogurt, salmon, sardines (with bones), molasses, broccoli, kale, and collard greens are good sources of calcium, but it's very difficult to get enough of this mineral through food alone. I recommend taking 1500 mg. of calcium daily along with 400 IU of vitamin D (to enhance absorption) and 500 mg. of magnesium. Do not drink colas that contain phosphate—they literally wash the calcium out of your body. Omega 3 fatty acids, which are available in capsules, are also essential for bone health.

Eating more soy foods can also help ease the transition to menopause in several important ways. First, soy foods such as tofu, tempeh, miso soup, and soy milk contain estrogenlike compounds, which can help relieve menopausal symptoms. Keep in mind that in Japan, where soy is a mainstay of the diet, there is no word for hot flash! Another reason to eat more soy: unlike synthetic forms of estrogen, these plant estrogens may actually help prevent breast cancer. (See the next question!) In addition, soy also helps to maintain bone, and protect against heart disease. If you don't eat soy foods, soy isoflavone extracts are available in tablets.

Finally, there are many herbal combination formulas on the market designed for menopausal women. Typically, they contain several herbs including red clover, licorice, dong quai, and vitex. Some of these formulas may work well for you. If you have untreated high blood pressure, avoid products containing licorice.

▓ Breast Cancer

Breast cancer runs in my family. Recently, I heard about a book that claims that diet and supplements can prevent breast cancer. Are there herbs that I should be taking?

Your risk of developing cancer is based on a combination of factors including genetics, lifestyle, and other unknown variables. Whether diet and supplements play a role in reducing the risk of developing cancer is controversial. What isn't controversial is the indisputable fact that, in certain parts of the world, breast cancer is a rare disease, but in the United States and other western countries, it is an epidemic. Mortality from breast cancer is significantly lower in Asian countries, notably where soy foods are routinely consumed in lieu of other forms of protein. It is highest in the west with our standard meat-and-potatoes diet. Given the fact that we know that soy contains many cancer-fighting compounds, including phytoestrogens called *isoflavones,* it seems reasonable to conclude that eating soy may help protect against cancer. That is why I recommend it in my book, *Earl Mindell's Soy Miracle,* and that is why I am in favor of taking soy isoflavone supplements if you do not regularly eat soy foods, such as tofu, or drink soy milk.

A diet rich in fruits and vegetables, especially cruciferous vegetables, such as broccoli, has also been linked to lower levels of breast cancer. These foods contain chemicals that, in test tube studies, have been shown to inhibit the growth of breast tumor cells.

Omega 3 fatty acids also show promise as cancer fighters. In animal studies, omega 3 fatty acids (found in salmon, tuna, and so on) have actually shrunk cancerous mammary tumors. Since omega 3 fatty acids are good for so many other things, it's advisable to include them in your diet.

Getting enough exercise, not smoking, and taking care of yourself in other ways will enhance your overall health and may also reduce the risk of breast cancer. It is equally important to get a mammogram every year and to see your doctor at the first sign of a problem. Early diagnosis is the key to long term survival.

Premenstrual Syndrome (PMS)

*About ten days before my period is due, I suffer from terrible PMS.
I get very cranky, my breasts become very sore, and I feel exhausted. Is there anything that can help?*

You're not alone. As many as 50 percent of all women may experience some form of premenstrual syndrome, including excessive water retention, headaches, mood swings, and breast tenderness. PMS disappears soon after menstruation begins. For some women, the symptoms are very minor and can be ignored. For other women, however, this is not the case, and like you, they spend a week or more each month in great discomfort. For these women, I recommend evening primrose oil. Several carefully conducted studies performed in London and Canada of women with severe PMS show that the majority of women studied experienced a marked reduction in symptoms after being treated with evening primrose oil. For best results, take between 500 to 1,000 mg. daily. It works well in combination with 400 IU of natural vitamin E (mixed tocopherols preferred).

Vitex is another popular treatment for PMS. Also known as *chasteberry*, vitex was once used in monasteries to reduce sexual desire. It probably works by controlling levels of the hormone prolactin, which can trigger PMS symptoms. Obviously, if you already have a low sex drive, avoid this herb! Vitex is available in tea or capsules. Take 20 mg. daily. In addition, during the time of the month that you are most vulnerable to retaining water, avoid salty food. Try eating herbs with natural diuretic properties such as alfalfa, asparagus, celery, dandelion, and carrot. Avoid excess caffeine, which could make you jittery. End the day with a relaxing cup of chamomile tea. You should notice a difference in how you feel almost immediately.

Regulating Menstruation After Birth-Control Pills

I've been taking birth-control pills for five years and now want to stop. I understand that it could take several months for my menstrual cycle to return to normal, and I'm worried about getting pregnant and not knowing it. Is there any herb that I should be taking during this transition period to promote normal menstruation?

You really should consult a well-informed physician or natural healer. In particular, use appropriate contraception if you do not want to get pregnant. Women herbalists recommend dong quai to help restore normal hormonal patterns in women who have taken birth-control pills. This herb, however, should not be used during pregnancy, or if you have excessive menstrual flow.

Menstrual Cramps

I suffer from bad menstrual cramps and am allergic to ibuprofen, the drug usually prescribed by doctors for this problem. Are there any herbal alternatives?

Fortunately, you have several excellent herbal options. Valerian, nature's own tranquilizer, can also help relieve uterine cramping. It is available in tea, extract, and capsules. Use valerian *only* at night. For cramping and headache, try white-willow capsules, a pain reliever similar to aspirin but less irritating to the stomach. In addition, many herb manufacturers have special formulas in capsule form designed to relieve menstrual cramps. Chamomile tea is an age-old remedy for cramping. Try one or more of these herbs to see which works the best for you.

Chronic Yeast Infections

I suffer from a recurrent vaginal yeast infection that is quite annoying. When I have an active case, I use an over-the-counter

cream that works right away to relieve the itchiness and discom-
fort but, a month or two later, the infection is back. Do you have
any suggestions?

Yeast is actually a minute fungus, and one of the stubbornest to control. There are some herbs with antifungal properties that can help. Start by taking oregano oil, which is not only a natural antiseptic, but contains compounds that can inhibit the growth of *candida albicans,* the primary cause of yeast infection. (For an active yeast infection, take six capsules daily for at least a month.) Pau d'arco, a South American herb, has been used fully against parasites and is lethal to fungus. Pau d'arco is also available in capsules. For centuries, women have used a douche made of goldenseal to cure all kinds of vaginal infections, including yeast. It's certainly worth a try. Goldenseal should not be used during pregnancy. Finally, build up your body's natural defenses against yeast infection by taking probiotics, supplements containing "good bacteria," which help to control the growth of yeast. Take 3 capsules (containing billions of organisms) daily. Take odorless garlic capsules daily to help prevent a recurrence.

Restless-Leg Syndrome

My legs are driving me crazy! When I'm sitting still, they feel
achy and stiff. As a result, I am constantly squirming and moving
around. My doctor called it restless-leg syndrome *and told me*
that it is quite common among women. He had no other advice to
give. Is there anything I can do about it?

Restless-leg syndrome, also known as *heavy-leg syndrome,* is caused by poor circulation. Several European studies show that many women with this problem find relief from butcher's broom, an herb that is widely available in capsule and extract form. Popular in Europe for more than a decade, butcher's broom is developing a following in the United States.

Varicose Veins and Hemorrhoids

I'm a dental hygienist, and spend most of the day on my feet. Although I wear support hose, I am still bothered by varicose veins. The veins on my legs are swollen and sore, especially at night. Are there any herbs that I should be using?

Varicose veins are veins that have become swollen and enlarged. They occur more often in women than men, and frequently are a result of pregnancy. *Hemorrhoids* are swollen or varicose anal veins. Varicose veins are a sign of poor circulation. In your case, standing on your feet all day is allowing the blood to pool in your legs, resulting in the varicosity. There are several time-honored remedies that are quite popular in Europe. Butcher's broom, which is used to improve overall circulation, has been shown to greatly relieve both varicose veins and hemorrhoids. For hemorrhoids, it is available in suppository form. Horse chestnut is another herb that is very soothing to inflamed veins. Look for it in special products designed to use on hemorrhoids. Applied externally, witch hazel will help reduce some of the discomfort caused by varicose veins and hemorrhoids.

Morning Sickness

Since I became pregnant, I wake up every morning feeling nauseated. Sometimes I feel sick again late in the afternoon. I'm afraid to take any antinausea medication because I don't want to hurt the baby. Any suggestions?

You have a classic case of *morning sickness*, a misnomer because it can strike anytime during the day, especially when you're feeling fatigued. To get rid of that feeling, drink a cup of ginger-root tea or take 1 ginger tablet or capsule first thing in the morning. During the day, alternate between drinking ginger ale or ginger tea and peppermint tea. None of these simple remedies will hurt your baby, and you'll feel a whole lot better.

▨ Labor and Delivery

*I'm working with a midwife and would like to avoid taking
painkillers during labor and delivery. What did women do before
meperidine and epidurals?*

In the old days, before high-tech delivery rooms, women prepared for
labor on their own. Starting at about the eighth month, they would sip
several cups of raspberry tea throughout the day to tone their uterus for
labor. During labor, they used herbs such as pennyroyal, blue cohosh,
and raspberry leaves to promote uterine contractions. Although these
herbs may not have reduced the pain, they may have helped to expedite
labor, which is half the battle. Talk to your midwife about having an
"herbal delivery." These herbs may be helpful even if you decide to use
painkillers.

▨ Episiotomy

*I'm pregnant with my second child. During my first pregnancy,
the worst part of labor and delivery was the episiotomy. The procedure was painful enough, but what really bothered me was the
fact that it took forever to heal. If I have to have an episiotomy
again, is there anything I can do to hasten the healing process?*

An *episiotomy* is a surgical incision of the vulva to prevent tearing during the second stage of labor. I have heard from many women that the
pain from the episiotomy can linger for several weeks, and even
months. There is an herb that may help. According to a 1966 study in a
French obstetrical journal, extract of *gotu kola*—sometimes called *centella*—helped to promote healing after episiotomy. The study noted
that the women who used centella extract immediately after the procedure reported less pain and faster healing than those who had been
given standard medication. The doctors in the study said that, for best
results, centella should be used as early in the procedure as possible.

Gotu kola or centella extract is easily available in most health food stores or herb shops. Obviously, you'll need your doctor's cooperation, so talk to him or her about using centella ahead of time.

Nursing

I want to nurse my baby but am having trouble producing enough milk. What herbs are good for nursing mothers?

For centuries, dill and anise have been used to promote milk production in nursing mothers. In fact, a recent study shows that just the smell of anise promotes milk production in cows! For best results, steep 2 teaspoons dill seed in 1 warm cup water for 10 to 15 minutes. Take ½ cup 2 to 3 times a day. To use anise seed, mix 1 teaspoon in 1 cup warm water. Drink up to 3 times daily. While you are nursing, avoid highly spiced foods or those heavily seasoned with garlic—these foods may make your breast milk less palatable to your baby. Also, avoid taking medication unless it is specifically recommended by your doctor, because it could pass from the milk to your baby.

Female Tonics

Are there herbs that are beneficial to the female reproductive system? Are there such things as aphrodisiacs?

Ginseng, which is recommended for menopausal symptoms, is also used as a tonic for both sexes. I recommend it! Followers of Ayurvedic medicine, the traditional medicine of India, consider the herb *shatavari* to be a general female tonic. You will see it included in herbal formulas designed for menopause and general female health. *Damiana* is considered a sexual tonic for both men and women and is reputed to be an aphrodisiac, although there is no scientific evidence to back up this claim. In folk medicine, asparagus and artichokes are highly regarded as aphrodisiacs for both sexes. In fact, although people have talked about aphrodisiacs for centuries, there is no scientific evidence to prove that they really exist.

Anemia

Are there any herbs that can help prevent iron-deficiency anemia?

I would recommend two herbs—nettle and chives. They are both rich in vitamin C and iron, a perfect combination, since vitamin C facilitates the body's absorption of iron. Iron is essential for the formation of red blood cells. Chives should be eaten fresh, but fresh nettle can be dangerous. Therefore, stick to extract, capsules, or dried herb, which are perfectly safe in the recommended dose.

Ovarian Cancer

I recently read about an herb called taxol that was being touted as a cure for ovarian cancer. Can you tell me more about it?

Taxol is an extract of the Pacific yew tree. It is used often in combination with other drugs, for cases of ovarian cancer that do not respond to conventional treatment. It is not a "cure" for everybody, but has helped some.

Cystitis

Help! It seems that I am constantly battling urinary-tract infections. Is there anything I can do to prevent them?

Cystitis is a bacterial infection of the bladder usually caused by *E. coli*, which normally occurs in the intestine. As you probably know by now, if you have an active bladder infection, you must see your doctor. Typically, one or more antibiotics will be prescribed to knock out the infection. If untreated, these infections can spread to the kidneys, which can be dangerous. There are some things you can do, however, to reduce your risk of getting another infection. First, make cranberry juice or capsules a part of your daily life. Cranberries help flush harmful bacteria out from the urinary tract, and contain natural antibiotics, called *anthocyanisides*. Drink one glass of unsweetened cranberry juice daily or take one 400 mg. cranberry capsule with each meal. Eat blueberries—they are also a good source of anthocyanisides.

Drink at least eight glasses of water daily to wash out your system. Take *probiotic supplements,* which contain friendly bacteria that helps keep bad bacteria like *E coli* under control.

CHAPTER 7

A Man's Body

One of the biggest changes to occur in the past decade has been the growing recognition by men of the importance of health. The stoic macho man who suffers in silence and never worries about his health is a relic of the past. Men today are deeply concerned about diet, supplements, exercise, and staying sharp and strong. In fact, it's interesting to note that men have quit smoking in greater numbers than have women!

Here are some answers to questions that I am frequently asked by men about herbal remedies for common male concerns.

▇ Getting Pumped

Are there any safe herbal supplements that can enhance my workout and build muscle?

First, I want to caution you to steer clear of steroids. *Synthetic steroids* are potent drugs that have many serious side effects, including death. In teenage boys, these drugs can interfere with normal sexual development. Steroids also depress the immune system, which will leave you more vulnerable to infection. In addition, they can cause fluid retention, high blood pressure, and other serious medical problems. Although they may increase muscle mass, they do not increase strength. Many weightlifters who rely on steroids for their brawny appearance may deceive themselves into thinking that they are stronger than they are. As a result, they may routinely overexert themselves, which can result in serious injury. Steroids are simply not worth the risk.

There are several herbal supplements that have become popular with the gym set. *Cordyceps,* derived from a Chinese mushroom and popular with Chinese athletes, is purported to enhance both endurance and athletic performance. Also from China comes *ciwuja,* an herb that supposedly helps you work out harder and longer. The Indian herb *puncturevine,* also known as *tribulus,* is reputed to stimulate the production of testosterone, which should increase muscle. Bromelain can help speed recovery after a hard workout. Keep in mind that there is no magic pill that will make you fit and strong. When it comes down to it, you still have to do the requisite exercise, although these herbs may give you a bit of a boost. (If you have an enlarged prostate or prostate cancer, do not take any products that increase the level of testosterone, which could stimulate the growth of prostate cells.)

Prostate Trouble

I recently went to my doctor for a checkup because I have to urinate very frequently, especially at night. My doctor told me that I have an enlarged prostate, which he said was not very serious. In fact, he did not even offer any treatment. Are there any herbs that can help? Am I likely to get prostate cancer?

The *prostate* is a group of small glands that surrounds the urethra at the point where it leaves the bladder. Although we don't know exactly what the prostate does, it secretes a fluid that is believed to stimulate the movement of sperm after ejaculation. Nearly every man over forty-five has some form of prostate enlargement and, in most cases, it is a harmless condition and not related to cancer, so relax. However, due to its location near the urethra, a sufficiently enlarged prostate can cause urinary problems. Any change in urinary patterns should be brought to the attention of your doctor. If urine is not passing properly, there is a greater risk of kidney infection or cystitis.

If the flow of urine is blocked, treatment, including surgery, may be necessary. However, in most cases, an enlarged prostate is a benign, albeit annoying, condition. In fact, as in your case, you may be told to simply live with it. There are some herbs that are reputed to be good for prostate problems. In Germany, saw palmetto is a highly regarded treatment for mild prostate conditions, and is fast becoming popular in the United States. Take three 500 mg. capsules daily. Saw palmetto works well with pygeum, nettles, zinc, and beta sisosterol. Look for special formulas containing these ingredients. In addition, avoid caffeinated drinks and alcohol, and try not to drink too much liquid before going to bed. (Similar to the popular hair growth product Propecia—Proscar in lower dosage—saw palmetto helps to control potent forms of testosterone that can promote hair loss.) The same prostate health formula that I take daily could stimulate hair growth.

Given the fact that about 40,000 men die of prostate cancer each year, I believe it is a disease that all men should know about. Although we don't know precisely how to prevent prostate cancer, several studies indicate that diet can help reduce the risk. Adding a serving of soy foods to your diet daily (tofu, miso, tempeh, or soy milk) may help reduce the risk of getting prostate cancer. These foods contains hormonelike compounds that may help control stronger hormones within the body that trigger the growth of tumors. What's the evidence? First, in countries where soybeans are a dietary staple, like Japan, the mortality rate from prostate cancer is strikingly lower than it is in the west. Second, numerous test-tube and animal studies have confirmed that particular compounds found in soy can inhibit the growth of prostate-tumor cells. I know that man cannot live on soy alone; the good news is that he doesn't have to. One of America's favorite foods, pizza, is also on the list of foods that may prevent prostate cancer. Cooked tomato-based products, such as pizza sauce and other tomato sauces, contain a type of carotenoid, *lycopene,* which appear to block the growth of prostate tumors. Since lycopene is fat soluble, it is better absorbed when cooked and combined with a little fat, such as oil and cheese.

Persistent Fungal Infection

Since I've joined a gym, I have developed a chronic fungal infection on my feet. It is extremely uncomfortable. My doctor gave me some antifungal pills, but they made me very nauseated. Is there anything else I can do?

A *fungus* is a microscopic plantlike organism that likes to take up residence on the human body. It's not surprising that you developed this problem after joining a gym—you probably picked it up in the shower or in communal dressing areas. There are a few herbs that can help strengthen your resistance against fungal infections. Oregano oil is one of them. It's antibacterial, antifungal, and reduces inflammation. Take up to 6 capsules daily until the fungus is cured. Pau d'arco is another herb that may help. Studies show that this South American herb has antifungal, antiparasitic properties. Take 3 capsules daily. Garlic can also help your body ward off these troublesome pests. Take 1 to 3 odorless garlic capsules daily. To relieve the dry, itchy feeling, use an ointment containing tea tree oil, a natural fungicide. Keep your feet as dry as possible and change your socks often. Some herbalists recommend sprinkling a mixture of goldenseal powder and talcum powder on your feet to absorb moisture and kill the fungus. Fungal infections are very persistent, and it may take several weeks (or even months) before you get relief.

Premature Baldness

The men in my family tend to go bald at an early age. I'm thirty-five, still have a full head of hair, and want to keep it that way! Are there any herbs that can help prevent hair loss?

Before I get your hopes up, it's important to note that patterns of hair loss are largely determined by genetics. Therefore, there are few legitimate remedies for baldness. In some cases, a sluggish thyroid or other medical problem may trigger hair loss and, once treated, the condition will very often reverse itself. There are some herbs that are reputed to prevent signs of premature aging, such as baldness, but these claims have not been scientifically investigated. However, they're certainly worth a try. The Chinese swear that fo-ti, a popular Asian tonic herb, prevents gray hair and other signs of aging. Take 1 capsule up to 3 times daily. Herbalists also recommend massaging the scalp with an extract of rosemary at the first sign of hair loss. After the treatment, shampoo as usual. As noted earlier, saw palmetto, well known as an herb for prostate health, may also help stimulate hair growth.

Sexual Dysfunction

I've heard a lot about herbal aphrodisiacs and, I wonder, is there an herb that can help impotence?

Long before Viagra was a household name, the bark of the yohimbe tree has been used as a treatment for impotency in Africa. In fact, the prescription drug *yohimbine,* an extract of this herb, is recognized as a legitimate treatment for impotence in the United States. A weaker form of yohimbine called *yohimbe* is sold over the counter, and may not work as well. However, yohimbine is potentially toxic to the liver and can cause a sudden decline in blood pressure. Therefore, it should only be used under the supervision of a qualified physician, if at all. Anyone who is suffering from chronic impotence should consult a doctor. The problem could be physical in origin, such as poor blood flow to the penis, or it could be a result of excessive stress or other psychological factors. In either case, treatment may be necessary.

Poor circulation due to hardening of the arteries (*atherosclerosis*) is a primary cause of impotence. Not smoking and eating a low-fat diet rich in fruits and vegetables will help prevent atherosclerosis in the first place. At least one study has shown that the herb ginkgo biloba can help restore sexual function in men suffering from impotence due to poor blood flow. Like Viagra, ginkgo helps regulate nitric oxide, an important chemical in the body that, among its other jobs, controls blood flow and is essential for perceiving pleasure and pain. You may have heard of ginkgo as a brain booster; it works by improving blood flow to the brain. When it comes to sexual function, ginkgo also enhances blood flow to the penis much the same way. Although it has never been tested, I suspect that pine bark extract, which shares properties with ginkgo, would have a similar effect. Take 60 mg. of ginkgo or pine bark extract daily. Here's some good news: Viagra is counterindicated for people taking medication for heart disease, but herbs such as ginkgo and pine bark extract have been used safely on heart patients for centuries. If you have a potency problem and can't take Viagra, talk to your doctor about taking these herbs.

I'm developing a "beer belly" and I don't even drink beer! What can I do to slim down?

Midcenter obesity—the "beer belly"—is a typical male problem. Aerobic exercise is a great way to burn fat all over your body, including your stomach. A low-fat, high-fiber diet is essential for weight loss. A combination of the Chinese herb immature bitter orange, country mallow-leaf extract, and green-tea extract may enhance your weight loss efforts by turning up your metabolism to burn fat faster. The Ayurvedic herb gymnema sylvestre may also help reduce the urge to eat sugary, high-calorie foods.

Muscle Strains

I'm a weekend athlete who frequently wakes up on Monday morning with sore, aching muscles. Any suggestions?

Arnica ointment is excellent for overworked muscles. Follow the directions on the package. However, don't use it on broken skin, as it can be very irritating. Eucalyptus ointment can also help by promoting blood flow to the sore areas, producing a feeling of warmth. Use several times daily as needed. In addition, white-willow bark, an herbal aspirin substitute, can reduce pain and inflammation. Take 2 tablets every 3 to 4 hours, as needed.

■ After-shave Rash

I have sensitive skin. Frequently, after I shave, my face erupts in a tiny, red rash that is very annoying. Are there any herbal products that might help?

Witch hazel is very soothing for minor skin irritations. Splash it on immediately after shaving. Calendula ointment is also excellent for sore spots. Apply after shaving. In addition, use an aloe gel daily to help restore moisture and promote healing.

CHAPTER 8

Anti-Aging Herbs

In 1900, the average life span was around fifty years. Think about it—by those standards, by the time you turned twenty-five, you were middle-aged! In contrast, demographers project that children born in this century will live on average eight decades, and many will live well beyond that. In fact, the fastest-growing segment of the United States population consists of those seventy-five and over. Modern medicine and advanced technology have done a wonderful job in extending life: There is no doubt that vaccinations, antibiotics, and other high-tech interventions have added years to our lives. There is much to be done, however, to enhance the quality of those added years. Too many people spend their later years in poor health, shuttling from doctor to doctor. To my way of thinking, there is no point in extending life if those last decades are spent in poor mental and physical health. The good news is that it doesn't have to be that way. I have come to believe that most of the illnesses that have become associated with aging are not a result of the aging process, but of years of neglect. Our new understanding of herbal medicine can help us maintain our strength and vitality well into our later decades.

For more than five thousand years, herbal practitioners have understood the simple fact that diet and lifestyle can have a profound effect on health. Until very recently, doctors who espoused this philosophy were considered radical, or were dismissed as practitioners of holistic medicine. It has only been within the past decade that the medical profession grudgingly accepted the link between a high-fat diet and a host of ailments, including cancer and heart disease. It has only been within the past few years that leading cancer researchers have finally begun to investigate the possibility of using potent antitumor chemicals found in fruits and vegetables to prevent cancer. While the medical profession has been dragging its feet, natural healers have been using herbs to promote wellness and prevent disease. In my opinion, the combination of twenty-first century high-tech medicine with herbal medicine will create longer, happier, and more productive lives for everyone.

Here are some herbs that will help you maintain a strong, sleek, healthy body and an agile mind.

■ Staying Smart and Sharp

"Where did I put the car keys?"

"I'm embarrassed to say, I forgot your name."

Does this sound familiar? Do you feel as if you're not as sharp as you used to be? Are you having trouble concentrating? Does it take you a bit longer to learn new skills? Rest assured that you're in good company. After age fifty, there are subtle yet tangible changes in brain function that can be quite annoying. In particular, there is a loss in function in short-term memory, which is why we may forget a phone number or an appointment unless it is written down. These age-related changes in mental function are caused by a slowdown in the production of key chemicals in the brain, called *neurotransmitters,* which are involved in learning and memory. Poor health, poor diet, sleep deprivation, and even boredom can make the problem worse. (A word of warning: If you are taking medication for a health problem, it could be aggravating age-related mental decline. If you are confused, unusually irritable, or have severe problems concentrating, talk to your doctor.)

To counteract the effects of brain aging, try these herbs for a brain boost. Keep in mind that they don't work overnight; it may be several weeks before you can see any difference.

Ginkgo Biloba

Maintaining good cardiovascular health is not only essential for a healthy heart, but key to a healthy brain. Ginkgo helps to regulate *nitric oxide,* a chemical in the body which helps control the circulation of blood. When blood flow to the brain is impaired because of *atherosclerosis* (hardening of the arteries), mental function can be adversely affected. In fact, many cases of senility are not due to Alzheimer's disease, a common cause of dementia, but are rooted in poor blood flow due to atherosclerosis. Ginkgo can help improve the blood flow to the brain, which will help restore mental function. Several European studies have shown that ginkgo can enhance mental acuity in older people, and at least one major U.S. study reported that it could slow down the progress of Alzheimer's disease. In a recent German study, one group of elderly patients was given extract of ginkgo and another group was given a placebo. Those given ginkgo showed an improvement in mental reaction time and were more alert than those who took the placebo. Those who had the slowest mental reaction time prior to taking ginkgo showed the greatest improvement after being given the ginkgo extract.

Take at least 120 mg. ginkgo daily. (I recommend that you take gingko in combination with 400 IU of vitamin E, and other brain boosters including club moss, gotu kola, schizandra, DMAE (dimethylaminoethanol, a naturally occurring substance found in food that enhances brain function), phosphatidyl choline, inositol, and serine, to get the best effect.)

Club Moss

This herb contains huperzine A which, in animal studies, has been shown to enhance memory. What's interesting is the fact that club-moss tea is a traditional Chinese treatment for memory loss and diminished cognitive function. You can purchase the whole herb in capsules, or standardized extracts in natural food stores.

Gotu Kola or Brahmi

Used in both Chinese and Indian medicine, this herb is a time-honored treatment for both stress-related disorders and memory problems. There is an interesting link between these two seemingly unrelated ailments. When we are under stress, our bodies produce stress hormones that, over time, can be harmful to every organ of the body, including the brain. In fact, chronic exposure to stress hormones can destroy cells in the region of the brain responsible for memory! No wonder studies have shown that people who have had stressful lives have poorer cognitive function later in life than people who have not been exposed to unrelenting stress. It's interesting that ancient healers were aware of the connection between stress and memory long before it was acknowledged by science.

In animal studies, gotu kola has been shown to improve memory. Gotu kola contains antioxidant compounds, which help protect brain cells from free radical damage. The cumulative effect of decades of exposure to free radicals is believed to be a contributing factor to age related memory loss.

Gotu kola is found in special herbal formulas designed to boost brain function and is sold separately in capsules and extract.

Rosemary

This herb contains chemicals that help preserve the breakdown of acetylcholine in the brain. A deficiency in acetylcholine is believed to be a contributing factor to senility in general, and Alzheimer's disease in particular. Rosemary is also an important antioxidant, which can help protect cells from free-radical attack. Use fresh or dried rosemary in your cooking, or look for new rosemary capsules at your natural food store.

Herbs for a Healthy Heart

You can learn an enormous amount about how people live from how they die. In most countries of the western world—especially the United

States—heart disease is the leading cause of death. Granted, cancer is a close second, but, for most of the twentieth century and at least the early part of the twenty-first, heart disease is, and will remain, the number-one killer. With rare exceptions, heart disease is very much a disease rooted in lifestyle. Stress, cigarette smoking, a diet high in saturated fat (from animal and dairy products), and lack of exercise are the major culprits. When it comes to heart disease, there are no magic bullets to either prevent or treat the problem. If you want to avoid heart disease, you need to be aware of the behaviors and habits that cause the problem in the first place. There are some herbs that can help bolster your efforts to stay heart healthy. In addition to using some of these herbs, I recommend taking 500 IU of vitamin E (dry succinate form) and 400 mcg. of folic acid.

Hawthorne

Earlier, I noted that, as we age, our brains begin to show particular age-related changes that we experience as a loss of short-term memory. Our hearts also begin to slow down, but the effects are not as sudden or obvious. Gradually, the heart loses some of its pumping action, which means that it does not circulate blood as effectively as it once did. Hawthorne is a mild cardiotonic that can enhance the pumping action of the heart. In Germany, it is routinely prescribed to older patients who don't need the more powerful drug digitalis, but nevertheless require some additional help. Hawthorne also improves the flow of blood to the heart and reduces blood pressure. Take up to two 200 mg. capsules daily. (To maintain a strong heart, I take a combination capsule of hawthorne, grapeseed and decaffeinated green-tea extract, mixed tocopherol, cayenne pepper, and Co Q10 twice daily.)

Grapeseed Extract

For thousands of years, wine has been used for medicinal purposes, but only recently have we learned that many of the benefits derived from wine can be found in grapeseed. Growing in popularity by leaps and bounds, grapeseed extract contains powerful compounds called *bioflavonoids,* which are potent antioxidants. Grapeseed extract helps prevent heart disease in several important ways. First, the antioxidants in grapeseed extract can protect LDL, or bad, cholesterol from oxidation. High levels of oxidized LDL cholesterol are believed to be a major factor in the formation of fatty deposits, called *plaque*, that lead to hardening of the arteries. Second, flavonoids work synergistically with vitamin C to strengthen capillaries, the smallest blood vessels, which helps promote good circulation. Flavonoids are also natural anti-inflammatories, not only helpful for conditions such as arthritis, but can also help prevent inflammation in blood vessels that can lead to hardening of the arteries. Take two 30 mg tablets of grapeseed extract daily. But don't stop eating grapes! Grape skins contain special compounds that are also beneficial to your heart.

Red Yeast

If you have been diagnosed with high cholesterol and triglyceride levels, this time-honored Chinese remedy may be just what the doctor ordered. It not only effectively cuts bad cholesterol levels, but reduces triglycerides, reducing your risk of both heart attack and stroke. Similar to prescription lipid-lowering drugs, red yeast should be avoided by anyone who has a liver problem or who drinks heavily. In fact, it is best to use this herbal supplement under the supervision of your physician, who should also be providing information on diet and exercise. The average dose is two 600 mg. capsules twice daily.

Green-Tea Extract

Popular in Asia, green tea is a more lightly processed form of the black tea that is favored in the west. Green tea contains flavonoids called *polyphenols*, which may be more powerful antioxidants than even vitamins C and E. (Although all forms of tea contain flavonoids, the kind found in green tea are believed to be especially beneficial.) Numerous studies confirm that people who drink all varieties of tea have a much lower incidence of heart disease than those who don't. According to a major study conducted in the Netherlands, men who drank the most tea, and consumed the highest amount of flavonoids in their daily diet, had a much lower risk of a fatal heart attack than those who did not.

The polyphenols in green tea are believed to prevent the oxidation of LDL cholesterol. You can either drink your tea or take green-tea extract tablets. I prefer green-tea extract that has been decaffeinated.

Flaxseed Oil

Thousands of years ago, our hunter-gatherer ancestors used to graze on flax along with other wild grasses. Our modern diet—highly processed and packed with convenience foods—is drastically different and deficient in many key nutrients. For example, flaxseed is an excellent source of omega 3 fatty acids, "good" fats often missing from the average western diet. Omega 3 fatty acids have been shown to lower overall cholesterol, reduce triglycerides, and prevent blood clots. Some studies suggest that omega 3 fatty acids can reduce blood levels of the protein homocysteine, which if elevated, can increase the risk of heart disease and stroke. As you will see in my section on cancer, this good fat also appears to protect against various forms of cancer. So, what are you waiting for? It's easy to get additional omega 3 fatty acids in your diet by taking flaxseed oil supplements. Flaxseed oil is sold in the refrigerator section of your natural food store, or in capsules on the shelves. Take 2 tablespoons oil daily, or two 1000 mg. capsules daily.

Guggul

If you lived in India and suffered from poor blood lipids, your Ayurvedic healer would recommend guggul as part of your daily treatment regimen. Indian studies show that guggul can reduce high cholesterol and triglyceride levels, helping to protect against heart disease and stroke. What's even better is that guggul does not appear to have many of the unpleasant side effects of conventional cholesterol-lowering drugs, such as upset stomach, nausea, and possible liver damage. It can also increase HDL. Take one 500 mg. standardized guggul capsule daily.

Turmeric

Some cuisines are just naturally heart healthy. One that quickly comes to mind is the cuisine of India, which includes many dishes seasoned with curry powder, a combination of fat-busting, antioxidant herbs that keep arteries clean. Turmeric is the herb in curry that gives it its yellow color. Turmeric cuts cholesterol levels by stimulating the production of bile by the liver, which uses up excess cholesterol. It is also a natural blood thinner, which prevents the formation of clots that can cause heart attacks. Turmeric is available in capsules. Take one to three capsules daily.

Soybean

Japan has the lowest mortality rate for heart disease for men in the world, and the second lowest for women. But, when Japanese men move to the United States, within a short time they are every bit as vulnerable to developing heart disease as Americans. Clearly, there's something that protects Japanese in Japan against heart disease that they lose when they leave their native country. Simply, it's their diet. Until the recent invasion of western-style fast-food restaurants in Japan, the typical Japanese diet consisted primarily of vegetables, rice, fish, and soybeans in various forms ranging from tofu to tempeh to miso. In fact, soybean is a mainstay of the Japanese diet. Not so coincidentally, soybeans contain many important compounds that protect against heart disease. First, they contain natural antioxidants that prevent free radical damage that can lead to elevated levels of bad cholesterol and damage to the heart muscle itself. Second, soybean protein has been shown to lower blood-cholesterol levels in both animals and humans. Third, *genistein,* a compound found in soy, appears to block an enzyme that promotes cell growth and migration that is believed to stimulate the formation of plaque deposits in arteries. It's easy enough to add soy to your diet but, for those of you who do not eat soy consistently, I recommend taking soy isoflavone supplements or drinking a soy-food beverage daily.

■ Type II Diabetes or Insulin Resistance

Diabetes refers to a group of biochemical disorders characterized by the body's inability to use *carbohydrates,* the sugars and starches that are found in food. The two most common types of diabetes are Type I and

Type II. Type I or juvenile diabetes strikes during childhood, and is caused by the failure of the pancreas to produce enough *insulin*, the hormone that breaks down glucose or sugar so it can be utilized by the body. Type II diabetes or adult onset diabetes is not caused by an inadequate supply of insulin, but rather by cells that have become insulin resistant. In either case, the end result is an elevated blood-sugar level that slowly destroys proteins in the body, causing serious damage to tissues and organs. As the disease progresses, complications arising from diabetes include permanent nerve damage, kidney damage, heart disease and blindness.

Type II diabetes is a virtual epidemic in the western world. In the United States, there are 16 million people with this form of diabetes, and an estimated one in four adults who are genetically predetermined to develop it. Since Type II diabetes strikes later in life, as baby boomers reach their fifth and sixth decade, the number of people with this disease is expected to rise exponentially. In fact, a seventy-year-old is twenty times more likely to become diabetic as a fifty-year-old. Diabetes is not inevitable. Positive changes in lifestyle and diet can make a huge difference in whether or not you will become diabetic. Obesity and a sedentary lifestyle are major risk factors for diabetes. If you are overweight, simply losing weight and becoming more active can substantially decrease your risk of getting this disease. Since sugar promotes the formation of troublesome free radicals, a high intake of antioxidant foods and supplements can also help keep diabetes at bay. Eating lots of fresh fruits and vegetables, avoiding processed, highly sugared foods, and adding two fatty fish meals a week to your diet can slash the risk of the disease. Foods such as legumes (soybeans, lentils, black beans, and so on), which are broken down slowly by the body, are excellent choices because they help prevent a sudden spike of sugar that can overwhelm the body's metabolic machinery. By the way, avoid soda—a recent study showed that women who drank the most soda were the most likely to develop insulin resistance. As any health-conscious person knows, smoking will only add to your problems. In the case of diabetes, it will speed up nerve damage. In addition, I recommend taking 400 IU of vitamin E (dry succinate form) daily. Also, daily take up to three 200 mcg. capsules of chromium picolinate, 500 mg. magnesium, and 50 mg. lipoic acid. Here are some herbs that can also help keep sugar under control. (If you are under treatment for diabetes or taking medication, work with your physician to incorporate herbs and diet into your treatment.)

Flaxseed Oil

A Dutch study showed that those who eat fish were less likely to develop *glucose intolerance,* a prediabetic condition, than those who don't. Only a small amount of fish daily (on average, 1 ounce) was all it took to reduce the risk. Fish contains omega 3 fatty acids, also found in abundance in flaxseed oil. Take two 1000 mg. capsules daily or two tablespoons of flaxseed oil. Store oil in the refrigerator.

Curry

Curry powder is a mix of spices that are rich in chromium, a mineral that can help control blood sugar. Curry is also delicious, a wonderful way to eat well and wisely. Curry is terrific with chicken, vegetables, and fish.

Gymnema Sylvestre

Ayurvedic healers use this herb as a treatment for diabetes. Known as the *sugar killer,* it is also believed to reduce the desire for sweet foods. Take two 200 mg. capsules daily.

Bitter Melon

Used in both traditional Chinese and Indian medicine, studies have shown that this herb can help normalize blood-sugar levels in Type II diabetes. One half hour before each meal, take one 500 mg. capsule.

Garlic

Animal studies have shown that compounds found in garlic can help lower blood-sugar levels. Since fresh garlic is so delicious, I recommend using it often as a seasoning. Garlic capsules are also available. Take one aged, odorless garlic 200 mg. capsule daily.

■ Protect Your Vision

There is nothing that can interfere with lifestyle as we age more than the loss of vision. There are two kinds of vision problems that are most common among older people: cataracts and macular degeneration. A *cataract* is a clouding of the lens that prevents light from reaching the pupil. A cataract can distort vision by making images appear vague and fuzzy. Cataracts are caused by constant exposure to sunlight, generating free radicals that destroy healthy tissue. Cataracts are so common that, if you live long enough, you will probably develop one! If untreated, a cataract can lead to blindness.

Macular degeneration, the leading cause of irreversible blindness in people over sixty, is also caused, if not aggravated by, free radicals. The macula is a small dimple on the retina that is responsible for fine vision. Damage to the macula can severely impair the ability to see and to perform basic tasks such as reading, writing, and driving.

Maintaining a healthy lifestyle can help maintain your vision. Smokers have a higher risk of both cataracts and macular degeneration: The message is, don't smoke. Eating a diet rich in antioxidants from fruits and vegetables can also help decrease the odds of developing these problems. Vitamins C and E in food and supplements should also help. A high-fat diet, which can clog arteries and hamper blood circulation to the eyes, can increase the risk of macular degeneration. I also recommend wearing sunglasses that block both UVA and UVB rays during peak sunlight hours. The following herbs may also help keep your vision.

Marigold

Marigold is rich in *lutein,* a member of the carotenoid family that is not only found in yellow fruits and vegetables, but in high concentration in the macula of the eye. Researchers suspect that it is there to protect against free radicals. Marigold, or lutein extracted from marigold, is available in many herbal formulas designed to protect vision. It is often combined with *zeathanthin,* another carotenoid found in the macula. Studies have shown that people who consume foods rich in lutein and zeathanthin have a significantly lower incidence of macular degeneration than those who do not.

Bilberry

Bilberry contains *anthocyanisides,* antioxidants that help protect microcirculation to the eyes. Anthocyanisides also help to regenerate *retinal pigment,* which helps the eye adapt to light. Take three 500 mg. capsules daily.

Amalaki

Rich in vitamin C, this Ayurvedic herb is prescribed to treat vision problems. The high vitamin C content helps quench free radicals before they can destroy the lens and macula of the eye. Look for amalaki in Ayurvedic anti-aging formulas.

Strong Body, Strong Bones

About half of all men and women over fifty will develop *osteoporosis,* a condition characterized by the thinning and weakening of bone, making them vulnerable to broken bones. Osteoporosis is very much a disease of aging. When we are young, we make new bone as we need it but, as we age, we use up more bone than we can replace.

Smoking and heavy drinking (more than two alcoholic beverages daily) can accelerate bone loss. A diet heavy in saturated fats, soda, and caffeine can also leach important minerals from the body, including calcium and magnesium, essential for the formation of new bone. On the other hand, a diet rich in low-fat dairy products, soy foods, fruits, and vegetables, and regular weight-bearing exercise (such as walking, weight lifting, tennis, and low-impact aerobics), help preserve bone. In addition to the herbs that I recommend here, take 1500 mg. calcium daily with 400 IU vitamin D, and 500 mg. magnesium daily.

Soy Isoflavones

A decline in key hormones, such as estrogen, is believed to be a major factor in the inability of old bones to repair themselves as efficiently as young bones. Recent studies suggest that estrogenlike compounds found in soy—*isoflavones*—can help maintain bone-building calcium and reduce bone loss. I take a combination tablet containing soy isoflavones, calcium, magnesium, vitamin D, and another mineral, boron, to stem bone loss. Look for soy isoflavones in herbal preparations designed to prevent osteoporosis.

Grapeseed and Green-Tea Extract

Grapeseed and green tea contain flavonoids, which help maintain *collagen,* an important component in bone. I use a combination product, but you can also take these herbs separately. Green tea is available in tea bags or tablets. Grapeseed extract is sold in capsules or tablets. (One green-tea extract tablet is equal to $1^1/_2$ cups green tea.) Take 100 mg. grapeseed extract twice daily.

Flaxseed Oil

The omega 3 fatty acids in flaxseed oil can help retain calcium, essential for strong bones. Finally convinced? If you're not taking flaxseed oil, you should be!

■ Sexual Rejuvenators

I've said it before and I'll say it again: Maintaining a strong healthy body is the best way to having a satisfying sex life, at any age. All of the supplements I recommend in this section will help preserve health, which is a key ingredient for a happy, fulfilled life. Obviously, fatigue due to illness, an aching body, or a depressed mind is not conducive to an active sex life. Unhealthy habits such as smoking, poor diet, and a lack of exercise can also create an environment that will hurt your ability to maintain a sexual relationship. Keep yourself vital and strong and a good sex life will follow. Frankly, I am wary of herbs that promise to restore sex drive or sexual function—there are few studies to either confirm or disprove these claims. However, if you are interested, here are some you can try.

Avena Sativa

Derived from the wild oat plant, this herb is reputed to rev up libido in both men and women. My advice is to try it and see if it works for you. Take 1 to 3 capsules daily.

Guarana

This South American herb has gained a reputation as a sexual stimulant, although I'm not sure why. Similar to the coffee bean, it is a source of caffeine. Perhaps it gained its reputation because it keeps you from nodding out before a romantic night. Keep in mind that, like strong coffee, guarana can be a stimulant and may interfere with sleep. Take up to three 500 mg. capsules daily.

Damiana

This herb is the aphrodisiac of choice in Central America. Natural healers prescribe it to men as a treatment for urinary-tract infections. Damiana is supposed to be a mild stimulant for men and women. Take one 60 mg. capsule up to three times daily.

Ginkgo Biloba

Similar to Viagra, ginkgo biloba can improve circulation to the genital areas in both men and women and, in studies of men, has been shown to enhance sexual performance. Unlike Viagra, which works almost immediately, ginkgo's effects may take several weeks to kick in. It may be well worth the wait—there are no dangerous side effects! Take two 60 mg. tablets daily.

Immune Boosters

When it comes to aging, we tend to focus on the more noticeable aspects, such as wrinkles and gray hair. What we forget is that some of the most profound changes are occurring quietly and insidiously inside our bodies. The impact of aging on the immune system is a case in point. As we age, there are some striking changes that occur in the immune system that can have a decidedly negative impact on our health. Our disease-fighting T-cells lose some of their strength, which leaves us vulnerable to infection. The same cold we could easily have shaken off in our youth stays with us longer when we are in our sixties, and beyond, and may turn into a more serious infection. That is why flu shots are routinely recommended for people over sixty. Our cancer fighting NK (*natural killer*) cells become sloppy, and allow cancerous growths to take hold, which is why the cancer rate rises exponentially with age. At the same time that our immune system has a weakened defense network against real threats, for reasons not fully understood, it often begins to attack our own "friendly" tissue, resulting in autoimmune problems, such as rheumatoid arthritis. The overall decline in immune function is called *immunosenescence.*

Immunosenescence is not inevitable: There are many things we can do to maintain a strong, functioning immune system. Diet and lifestyle play a major role. Deficiencies of key nutrients, such as antioxidant vitamins C and E, selenium, zinc, and vitamin B 6 can dampen immune function in older people. It is often difficult to get enough nutrients from food alone, which is why I feel it is so important to take the appropriate supplements. Lack of sleep can also inhibit the activity of important immune cells. Mild exercise can boost immune function, but don't overdo it—an overzealous workout that leaves you exhausted can deplete your immune system.

There are herbs such as elderberry, American feverfew, and echinacea that are excellent immune stimulants, but work best when you are sick. Here are two herbs that you can take when you are well to give you an added immune boost.

Pine-Bark Extract

In addition to the other wonderful things it does for you, pine-bark extract can help put some zip back into your immune system. Rich in flavonoids, this herb boosts the activity of another important immune-boosting antioxidant, vitamin C. Animal studies have shown that pine-bark extract can boost immune function in mouse models of both an HIVlike virus and alcoholism, two conditions that can seriously hamper normal immune function. Pine-bark extract also activates natural-killer cells that weed out cancer. Unlike other immune-stimulant herbs such as echinacea, which should only be used during times of illness, pine-bark extract is safe to take every day. The recommended dose is two 30 mg. capsules daily.

Barberry

Long before immunizations and antibiotics, ancient Egyptian healers used this herb to prevent plague. Ayurvedic healers still use it for intestinal upsets. Barberry contains *berberine*, which is believed to enhance immune function by stimulating immune cells called *macrophages*, white cells that circulate throughout the blood, gobbling bacteria, viruses, and other foreign invaders. Barberry has also been used in formulas to prevent cancer, notably the Hoxsey formula, which also included other herbs such as red clover. The nineteenth century eclectic physicians prescribed barberry for syphilis. Barberry should not be used during pregnancy or nursing. Barberry is often included in herbal formulas designed to stimulate immune function, along with other reputed herbal boosters like osha and astragalus.

Cancer-Fighting Herbs

Although we may not think of it as part of the aging process *per se*, cancer is very much a disease of aging. The chances of developing cancer rise exponentially with age. In fact, cancer is soon expected to surpass heart disease as the leading cause of death in the western world. I don't want to suggest that cancer is inevitable; it most certainly is not. You may be surprised to learn that the National Cancer Institute estimates that at least half of all cases of cancer are caused by environmental factors such as smoking, excessive alcohol intake, poor diet, and a sedentary lifestyle. In other words, you can substantially reduce your risk of getting cancer by making positive changes in your life. In fact, many of the same things that you should already be doing to prevent heart disease will also help stave off cancer. Eating lots of fresh fruits and vegetables, limiting your intake of saturated fat, and getting regular exercise will go a long way in keeping you heart healthy and cancer free. Simply not smoking and limiting your alcohol intake to no more than one or two drinks daily is another way to maintain your health. The good fat—omega 3 fatty acids—that I recommend to maintain heart health is also excellent for cancer prevention. Of course, when it comes to cancer, there are no guarantees. Genetics and other unknown factors may come into play, but it makes sense that maintaining a strong body will help reduce your risk. Here are some supplements that I believe can help tip the odds in your favor.

Broccoli Sprouts

New to supermarkets and natural food stores, broccoli sprouts are packed with more cancer-fighting compounds than full-grown broccoli. They're great in salads or eaten as a snack. As many of you know, broccoli contains several cancer-fighting compounds, including *indoles* which can deactivate carcinogens in the body. Indoles can also weaken potent estrogen that may stimulate the growth of various types of cancerous tumors. Broccoli also contains another important phytochemical—*sulforaphane*—which stimulates the body to produce cancer-fighting enzymes. According to the National Cancer Institute, only ten percent of all Americans eat the recommended five servings of fruits and vegetables daily needed to reduce their risk of cancer. Adding broccoli sprouts to your diet is an important step in the right direction.

Green Tea

Numerous studies show that green tea—the kind favored in Japan—may protect against many different types of cancer, including colon, lung, esophagus, pancreatic, and skin cancers. In a recent study, Japanese women who regularly drank green tea had a much lower risk of developing cancer than those who didn't. Green tea contains chemicals called polyphenols which some studies suggested are more powerful antioxidants than vitamins C and E. You can drink your tea, or take green tea extract. Drink it iced in the summer instead of colas or soft drinks! But steer clear of sugary prepared green tea beverages. They may not contain enough green tea to be effective.

Garlic

Since the days of Hippocrates, garlic has been held in high esteem for its cancer-fighting properties. Now science has caught up with the ancient healers. A recent study conducted in China found that those who ate the most garlic and other foods in the allium family, such as onions and chives, were least likely to develop stomach cancer. Garlic is believed to inhibit the formation of *carcinogenic nitrosamines,* which are made when additives in food are broken down by digestive juices. Researchers at Memorial Sloan-Kettering Cancer Center in New York City found that aged garlic could dramatically reduce the growth of prostate-cancer cells in test tube studies. I try to eat as much fresh garlic as possible, as well as taking a garlic supplement. I recommend one 500 mg. raw, aged, odorless garlic tablet or capsule daily. If you love garlic in your food but don't like garlic breath, eat a sprig of parsley to freshen your breath.

Soybean

Since *Earl Mindell's Soy Miracle* was published in 1995, I have been on a one-man crusade to get Americans to eat more soy foods. Why am I so passionate about soy? Study after study confirms that people who live in Asian countries, where soy is a dietary staple, have a dramatically reduced risk of dying of many different types of cancer than people who live in the west. In fact, if you live in the western world, your risk of dying of breast cancer or prostate cancer could be as much as ten to twenty times greater than if you lived in an Asian country! Soy foods contain an arsenal of cancer-fighting compounds, many of which protect against the effect of potent hormones in the body. I have incorporated tofu, miso soup, tempeh, veggie burgers, and soy milk into my diet. If you don't eat enough soy foods, consider taking a soy isoflavone supplement. You can drink a soy shake daily or take soy isoflavone supplement. (Be sure it contains two important phytochemicals, daidzein and genistein.)

Asian Mushrooms
(Reishi, Maitake, Shiitake)

Not only are they delicious, but many common varieties of Asian mushrooms contain potent cancer fighters. In particular, these mushrooms can help the body destroy cancer cells by boosting the immune system. Compounds derived from mushrooms are used in Japan as cancer treatments. Mushroom extracts are available in capsule or tablets, but I recommend adding these wonderful foods to your diet. They're great in soups, pasta, and as a topping on your favorite veggie burger. For a fabulous-tasting, cancer-fighting treat, make a pasta sauce with grilled shiitake mushrooms and sauteed broccoli in garlic and olive oil. You won't miss the cream and cheese!

CHAPTER 9

Looking Good

Whether you're a man or a woman, looking good goes hand in hand with feeling good. Before you read this chapter, however, I must caution that there is nothing on earth that can mask the ravages of an unhealthy lifestyle. The results of a lifetime of smoking, too much drinking, too little exercise, and a poor diet cannot be hidden under makeup or washed away by a scrub. Proper nutrition, the right vitamins, regular exercise, and sufficient sleep are the most important ingredients for staying attractive. Drinking eight glasses of filtered water daily is essential for healthy skin. Once you're living right, herbal preparations can help keep you looking your best.

Herbal products can be found in popular shops such as The Body Shop, Origins, and Crabtree and Evelyn as well as in department stores and natural food stores. In fact, just about any herbal skin or hair product can be found in a packaged form. However, making your own can be fun. Best of all, you can tailor your grooming aids to suit your specific needs.

Herbs for Great Skin

Antioxidant Herbs to Prevent Skin Aging

Most of the common skin problems—from crow's feet to wrinkles to cancer—are caused by the cumulative damage inflicted by UVA and

UVB rays from the sun. Both kinds of UV rays stimulate the formation of free radicals, which injure both the outer and inner layers of skin. The result is not only tired, old-looking skin, but an increased risk of skin cancer. Antioxidant creams and gels can help protect the skin from free-radical assault. They also work in synergy with vitamin C helping to restore *collagen,* the tissue that provides the scaffolding beneath the outer layer of skin. Herbal skin-care products derived from pine bark, grapeseed and green tea can not only help keep skin looking more youthful, but may even offer protection against skin cancer. For added antioxidant protection, look for skin products that also contain high potency vitamin C and E.

Regimen for Dry, Itchy Skin

People with dry skin should avoid exposure to harsh soaps and detergents, which will further deplete the body of its natural, protective oils. Stick to unscented, superfatted soaps made from natural ingredients including cocoa butter, aloe, jojoba oil, and wheat-germ oil. Chamomile is also an excellent cleanser that will not dry out your skin. After showering or bathing, always use a moisturizer to avoid that dry, tight feeling. Aloe and jojoba products are good choices. During the cold months, moisturize twice daily. Don't forget to moisturize your skin from the inside out: Taking a flaxseed-oil supplement daily can also help restore natural oils to dry skin.

Irritated Skin

Chamomile has a calming effect on highly sensitive skin. Calendula (derived from marigold) is also good for minor skin irritations.

Chapped Hands

Many people suffer from chapped hands, especially in the winter. To avoid irritation, wear cotton-lined rubber gloves when you wash dishes or do other household chores. In addition, for an excellent, old-fashioned hand cream—the kind that kept your grandmother's hands silky soft—mix $\frac{1}{2}$ cup rose water with 1 cup glycerin. Store in a plastic or glass jar. Rub on hands as needed.

At-Home Herbal Steam Facial

For just a few dollars' worth of herbs, you can give yourself the kind of steam facial typical of the swanky spas. It's easy to do, very relaxing, and a great way to deep-clean clogged pores. Boil 1 quart water. Mix in 2 tablespoons yarrow, 2 tablespoons lavender, 1 tablespoon peppermint, and 1 tablespoon fennel seeds. (Comfrey root, chamomile, and orange blossoms can be substituted for any of these ingredients.) Put pot in a low sink or on a table. Stand about 1 foot away. Make a tentlike cover out of a towel, and hold it over your head as you lean over the hot pot. Close your eyes. Let the hot steam penetrate your face. Take deep, relaxing breaths. After 5 minutes, pat dry. Apply moisturizer. Your skin will have a healthy glow.

Facial Scrubs

Although there are many different types of herbal facial scrubs on the market, they all do basically the same thing—they cleanse the skin by removing dirt, excess oil, and dead skin cells. Since most scrubs are slightly abrasive, they can be irritating to very sensitive skin. As a rule, they should not be used more than two or three times per week (and even less often if your skin is dry). There are many wonderful herbal scrubs on the market that include such traditional herbs as apricot, aloe, and almond. Some of the more exotic ones are worth a try. For example, I recently tried an exfoliating scrub made from sea kelp and herbs that was excellent. If you want to save money, it's very easy to make your own scrub. A handful of dried almond meal mixed in a little water does the job quite nicely. (Be sure to avoid getting the mixture in your eyes.) Rinse well and apply a moisturizer.

Herbal Facial Mask

A facial mask or peel eliminates the top layers of dead cells and also helps to tighten enlarged pores. It leaves the skin looking smooth and refreshed. There are several fine herbal products on the market, but it's easy enough to make your own mask with herbs that you probably have around the house. Mix 1 teaspoon peppermint leaves with 1 quart boiling water. Strain and save the water. To peppermint leaves, add 1 tablespoon dried almond meal and 1 tablespoon oatmeal. Add a few tablespoons water to make a thick paste. Apply to a clean face. Be sure to avoid your eyes. Wait until mask is dry (usually 15 minutes). Wash off with a warm washcloth. Your face will feel tingling and clean. Apply moisturizer.

Quick Facial Mask

Mash a fresh papaya and rub on clean face. Let dry. Remove with warm water and washcloth.

Terrific Herbal Skin Toner

For a quick pick-me-up, make an herbal skin freshener by mixing witch hazel with a splash of chamomile tea. When you need to feel (and look) revived, dab a small amount of this mixture on your face with a cotton ball.

Herbs for Beautiful Hair

Regimen for Dry Hair

Everybody wants strong, shiny, lustrous hair, but dry hair is often brittle and dull. A warm oil conditioner can help replenish some of the natural oils depleted by too much sun, hair dryers, and hair spray. This preparation is also an excellent dandruff treatment. Mix one cup extra-virgin olive oil (use a mildly scented, light oil) with 1/2 cup dried rosemary leaves. Warm on top of the stove in small pot. Remove from heat and let the mixture cool to a comfortable, warm temperature. Use a comb to separate your hair, and apply oil to dry scalp and hair with a cotton ball. Make sure to cover the entire scalp. Put a shower cap over your hair, and then cover with a turban made from a thin towel. Let the oil soak in for about 30 minutes. Wash out thoroughly with a mild, herbal shampoo. It will take several lathers to remove the oil. Do not use an additional conditioner—you won't need it. Repeat treatment monthly. Your hair will be shiny and more manageable.

Quick Rinse for Dry Hair

Brew 2 cups marshmallow tea. Let cool. Rinse through after shampoo.

Regimen for Oily Hair

Overzealous oil glands can leave hair stringy and limp. Horsetail (silica) is the herb to use to control excess oil production and to bring life back to listless, uncooperative hair. There are several commercial hair products available in health food stores that contain horsetail or silica.

Rinse to Bring Out Blond Highlights

Since the days of the Roman Empire, chamomile has been used to add golden highlights to light-colored hair. For an excellent highlighting rinse (that's good enough to drink) put 2 tablespoons dried chamomile into 16 ounces hot water. Simmer $\frac{1}{2}$ hour. Add the juice of 1 small lemon. After you shampoo, lean over the sink, and pour herbal mixture through hair slowly, making sure that the entire head of hair is covered. Catch remaining fluid in a bowl. Let mixture stand on hair 1 minute and then pour remaining fluid over hair. (Be sure to avoid your eyes; the lemon will make them sting.) Rinse out thoroughly with warm water. Repeat weekly. You'll notice a real difference in your hair, especially in the sunlight.

Rinse for Dark Hair

If you want to bring out a rich, dark sheen, try this recipe. Make 2 cups regular, dark tea. You can use a commercial teabag. Add 2 tablespoons dried rosemary leaves. Let simmer for 30 minutes. After you shampoo, lean over the sink, and pour herbal mixture through hair slowly, catching the remaining fluid in a bowl. Let mixture stay on hair for about a minute, and pour remaining fluid over hair. Massage mixture into hair. Rinse thoroughly with warm water. Repeat weekly.

Rinse to Rid Hair of Shampoo Residue

After shampooing, a vinegar rinse is the best way to wash out any shampoo buildup, which can make the hair look dull. Put $^1/_4$ cup dried rosemary and $^1/_2$ cup dried peppermint in a bowl and set aside. Put 2 cups clear apple-cider vinegar in a pot. Warm vinegar until it almost reaches boiling point. Pour vinegar over herbs. Let cool. Pour into a plastic container and let stand for one week, shaking daily. Strain mixture through a double layer of cheesecloth and add a few drops of a nicely scented essential oil to mask the vinegar smell. After washing your hair, mix $^1/_2$ cup herbal vinegar to 3 to 4 cups water, and pour mixture over hair as final rinse. Use weekly to avoid excess shampoo residue.

Don't Try This at Home!

Approximately 120 years ago, this homemade hair rinse was believed to promote hair growth.

- 3 quarts rum
- 1 pint "spirit of wine"
- 1 pint water
- $^1/_2$ ounce extract of catharides (Spanish fly)
- $^1/_2$ ounce carbonate of ammonia
- 1 ounce salt of tartar

Herbal Eye Care

Tired, worn-out–looking eyes can make you look old before your time. Fatigue, pollution, and allergies are all possible causes of red, sore eyes. To give tired eyes a lift, place fresh cucumber slices over each eye. Lie down in a dark room for 30 minutes. Your eyes will look and feel less sore and puffy. Beware of using commercial eye drops. Frequent use of these over-the-counter products can result in chronic eye irritation. If you need to use an eyewash, try eyebright. Mix 2 tablespoons of the herb in 16 ounces hot water. Let cool. Strain. Use a small cup to pour mixture into each eye, or apply to each eye with a clean cotton ball. Do not use the same cotton ball for both eyes, as this may spread the infection.

Herbs for Strong Nails

If your nails are constantly peeling and chipping, or if they have white spots, you need to include more calcium in your diet. Eat more broccoli, collard greens, and low-fat dairy products. In addition, take a horsetail (silica) supplement, which facilitates the absorption of calcium by the body.

If your nails are dry and splitting, and your cuticles are ragged, a hot oil treatment can be very beneficial. Warm 1/2 cup almond oil in a small pot. (Don't let it get too hot.) Pour into a bowl and soak the fingertips on each hand for about 15 minutes. Rub remaining oil into cuticles, hands, and on the soles of the feet for a smooth, satiny feeling.

CHAPTER 10

Aromatherapy

*"The way to health is to have an aromatic bath
and a scented massage every day."*

—H I P P O C R A T E S

Whenever *I get* a whiff of eucalyptus oil, it takes me back to my childhood in Canada. My family would go to a hotel that had a steam bath in the basement, where my father and I would trek periodically to cleanse our pores and inhale the fumes emitted from buckets full of fresh eucalyptus leaves floating in hot water. I'll never forget the effect of those leaves. My sinuses would clear, my thoughts would become sharper, and I would leave the steam bath feeling exhilarated.

Many years later, when I learned about aromatherapy, I understood the lure of those steam baths. The power of scent is the guiding principle behind aromatherapy: the use of scented oils to soothe, relax, and heal. In some cases, aromatherapy is also used to treat specific medical problems. Massaged into the skin, certain oils can relieve muscle aches and pains. Some oils are also strongly antiseptic. When an epidemic of plague broke out in ancient Athens, Hippocrates urged the people to burn aromatic plants on the street corners to prevent the plague from spreading. Even in those primitive times, the father of modern medicine somehow knew that the oils emitted by these plants were strong medicines. Centuries later, researchers in the Soviet Union discovered that *eucalyptus oil,* a powerful natural antiviral agent, was useful for treating certain strains of influenza.

Today, essential oils are usually used externally: They may be inhaled, rubbed into the skin, or used in the bath. They may also be taken internally (in a diluted form) as medicine, but only under the supervision of a qualified practitioner. A full-strength essential oil should never be taken orally—it can be very irritating.

One of the fastest-growing modes of alternative medicine, aromatherapy has been practiced since ancient times. The Egyptians rubbed cumin on their bodies prior to intercourse to promote conception. They also used strong oils in the embalming and mummification process, probably as disinfectants. Ancient Romans wore garlands of roses on their heads to cure headaches. Native Americans used the oil of the morning glory to prevent nightmares and prickly ash perfume to promote feelings of love.

Several scientific studies reinforce the therapeutic value of essential oils. For example, researchers at Milan University have successfully treated depression and anxiety using aerosol (sprayed) oils. Scientists in England have recently reported that lavender aromatherapy was as effective a sleep aid as sleeping pills for nursing-home patients with insomnia. Of course, unlike sleeping pills, there is no drug-induced morning-after hangover with lavender!

How does aromatherapy work? Once inhaled through the nose, the essential oils stimulated the olfactory organs, which are linked to the areas of the brain that control emotions. According to aromatherapists, when these essential oils are rubbed on the skin, they stimulate a reaction on the nerve endings on the skin's surface. This reaction passes through the nerves until it reaches the pituitary or master gland. In turn, through a series of chemical reactions, the pituitary controls whether we feel stressed or relaxed.

Different oils elicit different physical and emotional responses. Some calm us; some excite us. Some make us happy; some make us reflective. Some enhance our spiritual side; some increase our desire for carnal pleasures.

Essential oils can be purchased at herb shops and health food stores. They are very strong: a little goes a long way. Here are some tips on how to use essential oils:

- *Never inhale from the bottle directly. Rather, mix 1 or 2 drops into a bowl of steaming hot water. Place a towel over your head and around the bowl to catch the steam.*
- *If you want to use an essential oil in the bath, place 5 or 6 drops in the warm water.*
- *For massage, use 3 or 4 drops of the appropriate scented oil. Use only diluted essential oils designed specifically for use on the skin.*
- *Another safe way to get the benefit of essential oils is to put a few drops of oil in a special lamp called an aroma defuser, which is sold in herb shops.*

The following is a list of commonly used essential oils and the response they are believed to evoke.

Apple	Cheering
Basil	Promotes peace and happiness
Bay leaf	Increases psychic awareness
Benzoin	Promotes energy
Bergamot	Promotes restful sleep
Bergamot mint	Increases energy
Black pepper	Increases alertness
Broom	Promotes tranquility
Calendula	Promotes good health
Camphor	Increases energy
Caraway	Increases energy
Cardamom	Promotes feelings of love and desire for sex
Carnation	Increases energy
Catnip	Calms you down
Cedar	Increases spirituality
Celery	Promotes a restful sleep
Chamomile	Promotes sleep and tranquility
Cinnamon	Increases energy and awareness
Clove	Promotes healing
Coffee	Enhances the conscious mind
Coriander	Improves memory

Cumin	Immune booster
Cypress	Promotes healing
Daffodil	Increases feelings of love
Deer tongue	Promotes sexuality
Dill	Sharpens the conscious mind
Eucalyptus	Promotes healing
Fennel	Promotes longevity
Frankincense	Increases spirituality
Gardenia	Promotes feelings of peace and love
Garlic	Promotes health, purifies the body
Geranium	Promotes happiness
Ginger	Increases energy
Hops	Promotes sleep
Hyacinth	Helps to overcome grief
Hyssop	Purifies the body
Iris	Increases feelings of love
Jasmine	Promotes love, sex, and sleep
Juniper berry	Promotes healing
Lavender	Counteracts insomnia
Lemon	Promotes health, healing, and energy
Lemon grass	Purifies the body
Lemon verbena	Increases feelings of love
Lilac	Increases feelings of love
Lily	Promotes inner peace
Lily of the valley	Improves memory
Lime	Increases energy
Magnolia	Promotes feelings of love
Marjoram	Promotes sleep
Mimosa	Promotes psychic dreams
Myrrh	Promotes healing
Narcissus	Enhances feelings of love
Nutmeg	Increases energy
Onion	Immune booster

Orange	Increases joy and energy
Peppermint	Sharpens the conscious mind
Pine	Promotes healing
Rose	Promotes feelings of love and peace
Rosemary	Promotes longevity
Rue	Calms you down
Saffron	Increases energy
Sage	Improves memory
Sandalwood	Promotes healing and sexuality
Spearmint	Promotes healing
Star anise	Increases awareness
Sweet pea	Promotes happiness
Thyme	Promotes good health
Tulip	Purifies the body
Vanilla	Promotes sex and love
Water lily	Promotes peace and happiness
Wood aloe	Increases feelings of love
Yarrow	Increases awareness
Ylang ylang	Promotes sex and love

Selected Bibliography

"Aloe Vera: The Powerful Healing Herb." The Vitamin Connection 37–39, Nov./Dec. 1990.

al-Hindawi, M. K., al-Khafaji, S. H., and Abdul-Nabi, M. H. "Antigranuloma Activity of Iraqi Withania Somnifera." Journal of Ethnopharmacology 37, no. 2:113–116, 1992.

Austin, Frederick G. "Schistosoma Mansoni Chemoprohyiaxis with Dietary Lapachol." The American Journal of Tropical Medicine and Hygiene: 412–419. Vol 23, No. 3, 1974.

Blumenthal, Mark. "A Guide to Sedative Herbs." Health Food Business: 40–67, June 1990.

———. *"Herbal Update."* Whole Foods: 48, April 1991.

———. *"South American Herbs."* Health Foods Business: 52–53, February 1990.

Boericke, William. Pocket Manual of Homeopathic Materia Medica. *Philadelphia, PA: Boericke & Runyon, 1927.*

"Botanical Field Producing Hearty Growth Areas." Whole Foods: 46–98, November 1990.

"Botanicals Generally Recognized as Safe." Herb Research Foundation, Boulder, CO.

Botanical Research Summaries, Eclectic Dispensatory of Botanical Therapeutics. *Eclectic Institute, Portland, OR.*

Braeckman, J. "The Extract of Serenoa Repens in the Treatment of Benign Prostatic Hyperplasis: A Multicenter Open Study." Current Therapy Research 55:776–785, 1994.

Briggs, Colin J. "Evening Primrose: La Belie de Nuit, The King's Cureall." Canadian Pharmacy Journal 119 (5):249–252, 54, May 1986.

Brody, Jane E. "Personal Health: A Note of Caution in Exploring the World of Medicinal Herbs: It's a Jungle Out There." The New York Times: Feb. 15, 1990.

————. "Fortified Foods Could Fight Off Cancer." The New York Times: *February 19, 1991.*

Brown, Donald. *"Botanical Medicine in America: The Medical Connection."* Let's Live: *50–52, February 1990.*

Brown, L., Hankinson S. E., Seddon, J. M., et al. *"A Prospective Study of Carotenoid Intake and Cataracts Among U.S. men."* American Journal of Epidemiology. *147:S54 (Abs 213).*

Cameron, E. and Pauling, L. Cancer and Vitamin C. *Phil., Pa: Camino Books, 1993.*

"Capsules. (The Pacific Yew Tree.)" Pharmacy West: *30, January 1991.*

Carotenoid Fact Book. *La Grange, IL: 1996. VERIS Research Information Service.*

Carter, James P. *"Gamma-Linolenic Acid as a Nutrient."* Food Technology *42 (6):72, 74–75, 78–79, 81–82, June 1988.*

Castleman, Michael. *"Friend or Foe?"* (Comfrey) The Herb Quarterly *44:18–23, Winter 1989.*

————. *"An Herbal Remedy for Migraines."* The Herb Quarterly *43:8–1, Fall 1989.*

Chihal, Jane H. *"Premenstrual Syndrome: An Update for the Clinician."* Obstetrics and Gynecology Clinics of North America *17 (2): 457–479, June 1990.*

Cichoke, A. *"Maitake: The King of Mushrooms."* Townsend Letter for Doctors *130:432–433, May 1994.*

Colbin, Annemarie. Food and Healing. *New York: Ballantine Books, 1986.*

Combest, W. L., and Nemecz, G. *"Echinacea."* U.S. Pharmacist *22 vol. 10 126–132, 1997.*

Cousins, E., Lee, R., and Packer, L. *"ESR Studies of Vitamin C Regeneration, Order of Reactivity of Natural Source Photochemical Preparations."* Biochemistry and Molecular Biology International, *45:583–597. 1998.*

Crellin, John K., and Philpott, Jane. Herbal Medicine Past and Present, Volume 2. A Reference Guide to Medicinal Plants. *Durham: Duke University Press, 1990.*

Culpeper, Nicholas. Culpeper's Complete Herbal. *London: W. Foulsham & Co., Ltd.*

Dobelis, I., and Ferguson, G. Reader's Digest Magic and Medicine of Plants. *Pleasantville, NY: Reader's Digest Books, 1986.*

"Extract from Kudzu Vine Curbs Alcohol Desire; Diadzein and Daidzein." The Addiction Letter 9 no. 12, December 1993.

Farnsworth, Norman R., Akerele, O., et al. "Medicinal Plants in Therapy." Bulletin of the World Health Organization: 63 (6) 965–981, 1985.

Fox, Timothy R. "Aloe Vera: Revered, Mysterious Healer." Health Foods Business: 45–4, December 1990.

Gabriel, Ingrid. Herb Identifier and Handbook. New York: Sterling Publishing Company, 1979.

"Garlic Folk and Fact." Whole Foods: 75, January 1991.

Grandinetti, Deborah. Prevention: 48–50, December 1988.

Hassam, A. G. "The Role of Evening Primrose Oil in Nutrition and Disease." The Role of Fats in Human Nutrition. Chichester, England: Ellis Horwood, 1985.

Hashim, S., Aboobaker, Madhubala, R., et al. "Modulatory Effects of Essential Oils From Spices on the Formation of DNA Adduct by Aflatoxin B1 in Vitro." Nutrition and Cancer. 21:169–175, 1994.

Harrer, G., et al. "Treatment of Mild/Moderate Depressions With Hypericum." Phytomedicine 1:3–8, 1994.

Hausman, Patricia, and Hurley, Judith Benn. The Healing Foods: The Ultimate Authority on the Curative Power of Nutrition. Emmaus, PA: Rodale Press, 1989.

Hepinstal, S., et al. "Extracts of Feverfew Inhibit Granule Secretion in Blood Platelets and Polymorphonuclear Leucocytes." The Lancet: 1071–1073, May 11, 1985.

"Herb: Just Another 4-Letter Word for Drug." Longevity: 51–55, April 1991.

"Herbs for Healthy Skin and Hair." Whole Foods: 84, October 1990.

Heymsfield, S., Allison, D., Vasseli, J., et al. "Garcinia Cambogia (Hydroxycitric Acid) as a Potential Antiobesity Agent." JAMA 280–18, November 11, 1998.

"Origins of Nutrition and Diabetes." Nutrition Today: 13–18, Jan./Feb. 1991.

Hobbs, Christopher. "The Chaste Tree: Vitex agnus castus." Pharmacy in History 33 (1):19–22, 1991.

Holmes, Peter. The Energetics of Western Herbs: Integrating Western and Oriental Herbal Medicine Traditions. *Vol. 1. Boulder, CO: Artemis Press, 1989.*

Horrobin, David F., and Manku, Mehar S. *"Clinical Biochemistry of Essential Fatty Acids."* Omega 3 Essential Fatty Acids: Pathophysiology and Roles in Clinical Medicine. *Alan R. Liss, Inc: 21–53.*

Igram, Cass. The Cure Is in the Cupboard: How to Use Oregano for Better Health. *Knowledge House, New York, 1997.*

Kail, Konrad. *"Natural Stimulants."* Health Foods Business: *51–52, January 1991.*

Keller, K. L., and Fensje, N. A. *"Uses of Vitamins A,C and E and Related Compounds in Dermatology: A Review."* Journal of the Academy of Dermatology. *39:611–625, 1998.*

Kloss, Jethro. Back to Eden. *Loma Linda, CA: Back to Eden Publishing Company, 1936.*

Knekt, P., Jarvinen, R., Reunanen, A., et al. *"Flavonoid Intake and Coronary Mortality in Finland, a Cohort Study."* British Medical Journal *(Clincal Research Ed.) 312 (7029):478–481.*

Kronick, Jeff. *"New Ways of Looking at Herbs for Americans."* Whole Foods: *54–56, February 1990.*

"Oil of Evening Primrose." Lawrence Review of Natural Products. *March 1989.*

Le Bars, P. L., Katz, M. M., et al. *"A Placebo-Controlled, Double-Blind, Randomized Trial of an Extract of Ginkgo Biloba for Dementia."* North American EGb Study Group. JAMA *278 (16):1327–1332.*

Leung, Albert Y. *"The Proper Use of Herbs."* Whole Foods: *8183, November 1990.*

———. *"The Herbal News." 2: Fall 1990.*

Longcope, Christopher. *"Relationships of Estrogen to Breast Cancer, of Diet to Breast Cancer, and of Diet to Estradiol Metabolism."* Journal of the National Cancer Institute *82 (11), June 6, 1990.*

Leyel, C. F. Herbal Delights. *New York: Gramercy Publishing Company, 1938.*

Lucas, Richard. Common and Uncommon Uses of Herbs for Healthful Living. *West Nyack, NY: Parker Publishing Company, Inc., 1969.*

Lust, John. The Herb Book. *New York: Bantam Books, 1974.*

Mabley, Richard. The New Age Herbalist. *London: Gaia Books, 1988.*

Mars, Brigette. "Herbs to Know About During Pregnancy." Let's Live: 74–75, February 1991.

Matthew, B., and Sankaranarayanan, P. "Evaluation of Chemoprevention of Oral Cancer with Spirulina Fusiformis." Nutrition and Cancer 24 no. 2:198–202. 1995.

McCaleb, Rob. "What's New With Ginseng?" Herb Research Foundation, December 18, 1990.

Michnovicz, Jon, and Bradlow, H. Leon. "Induction of Estradiol Metabolism by Dietary Indole3-carbinol in Humans. Journal of the National Cancer Institute 82 (11), June 6, 1990.

Mindell, Earl. Earl Mindell's Vitamin Bible. New York: Warner Books, 1985.

————. Earl Mindell's Soy Miracle. New York: Fireside Press, 1995.

Mowry, Daniel B. Guaranteed Potency Herbs: Next Generation Herbal Medicine. New Canaan, CT: Keats Publishing Company, 1990.

————. The Scientific Validation of Herbal Medicine. New Canaan, Conn. Keats Publishing Company, 1994.

Murphy, J. J., Hepinstall, S., and Mitchell, J. R. A. "Randomized Double-Blind Placebo Controlled Trial of Feverfew in Migraine Prevention." The Lancet: 189–192. July 23, 1988.

Murty, N. Anjneya, and Pandey, D. P. Ayurvedic Cure for Common Diseases. New Delhi: Orient Paperbacks, 1982.

Packer, Lester, and Colman, Carol. The Antioxidant Miracle. New York: John Wiley and Sons, 1999.

Passwater, Richard A. "Antioxidant Nutrients and Heart Disease." Whole Foods: 49–52.

Peterson, Nicola. Culpeper Guides: Herbs and Health. London: Webb & Bower, 1989.

Privitera, James R. Olive Leaf Extract: A New/Old Healing Bonanza for Mankind. Corvina, CA: Nutrascreen, 1996.

Rice-Evans, C. and Packer, L. Flavonoids in Health and Disease. New York: Marcel Dekker, Inc., 1998.

Rose, Jeanne. Modern Herbal. New York: Perigee Books, 1987.

Ryman, Daniele. The Aromatherapy Handbook. Essex, England: The C. W. Daniel Company, Ltd., 1989.

Salmi, H. A., et al. "Effects of Silymarin on Chemical, Functional and Morphological Alternations of the Liver." Scandanavian Journal of Gastroenterology 17:517–521, 1982.

Santillo, Humbart. Natural Healing with Herbs. Prescott Valley, AZ: Hohm Press, 1984.

Shansugasundaram, E. R. B., et al. "Use of Gymnema Sylvestre Leaf Extract in the Control of Blood Glucose in Insulin-Dependent Diabetes Mellitus." Journal of Ethnopharmacology 30:281–294, 1990.

Shewell-Cooper, W. E. Plants, Flowers and Herbs of the Bible. New Canaan, CT: Keats Publishing, 1977.

Shibata, Shoji, Osamu, Tanaka, et al. "Chemistry and Pharmacology of Panax." Economic and Medicinal Plant Research 1:218284. London: Academic Press Inc., 1985.

Sikora, R., et al. "Ginkgo Biloba Extract in the Therapy of Erectile Dysfunction." Journal of Urology 141:141–188a, 1989.

Simopoulos, A. "Omega-3 Fatty Acids in Health and Disease and in Growth and Development." American Journal of Clinical Nutrition. 54:438–463, 1991.

Singh, Y. N. "Kava: An Overview." Journal of Ethnopharmacology 37, 1:13–45, 1992.

Smit, H. F., Woerdenbag, H. J., Singh, R. H., et al. "Ayurvedic Herbal Drugs with Possible Cytostatic Activity." Journal of Ethnopharmacology 47:75–84, 1995.

Stanway, Andrew. The Natural Family Doctor: The Comprehensive Self-Help Guide to Health and Natural Medicine. London: Gaia Books Ltd., 1987.

Stolzenburg, William. "Garlic Medicine: Cures in Cloves?" Science News: 157, Sept. 8, 1990.

Swenson, A. Allien. Your Biblical Garden: Plants of the Bible and How to Grow Them. Garden City, NY: Doubleday and Co., 1981.

Syed, T. A., et al. "Management of Psoriasis with Aloe Vera Extract in a Hydrophylic Cream: a Placebo Controlled-Double Study." Trop Medicine & Internal Health 1:505–509. 1996.

Teeguarden, Ron. Chinese Herbal Tonics. Tokyo: Japan Publications, 1984.

Teel, R. W., et al. "Antimutagenic Effects of Polyphenolic Compounds." Cancer Letter 66, no 2:107–23, September 30, 1992.

Tham, D. M., Gardner, C. D., and Haskell, W. L. "Potential Health Benefits of Dietary Phytoestrogens: a Review of Clinical, Epidemiological, and Mechanistic Evidence." Journal of Endocrinology and Metabolism 83:2223–2225, 1998.

"The Top Ten Herbs of the '90s." Health Food Business: 46–83, October 1989.

Tisserand, Robert. Aromatherapy: To Heal and Tend the Body. Santa Fe: Lotus Press, 1988.

Tobe, John H. Proven Herbal Remedies. Ontario, Canada: Provoker Press, 1969.

Tyler, Varro E. "Plant Drugs in the 21st Century." Economic Botany 40 (3):279–288, 1986.

"Up and Coming Herbs: A Look Toward the Herbal Horizon." Whole Foods: 24–26, April 1991.

Volz, H., and Kieser, M. "Kava-kava Extract WS 1980 versus Placebo in Anxiety Disorders—a Randomized Placebo Controlled 25 Week Out Patient Trial." Pharmocopsychiatry. 30:1–5, 1997.

"Vulnerable Yew Tree Yields Cancer Treatment." National Geographic, April 1991.

Wagner, H., Kikino, Hiroshi, and Farnsworth, Norman R. "Siberian Ginseng (Eleutherococcus senticosus): Current Status as an Adaptogen." Economic and Medicinal Plant Research, London: Academic Press, 1985.

Ward, Harold. Herbal Manual. London: The C.W. Daniel Company Ltd., 1936.

Weed, Susan S. Wise Woman Herbal Childbearing Year. Woodstock, NY: Ash Tree Publishing, 1986.

Weil, Andrew. "A New Look at Botanical Medicine." Whole Earth Review 64, Fall 1989.

Weiner, Michael. Herbs and Immunity. San Rafael, CA: Quantum Books, 1990.

————. "Native American Herbs: A New Look at a National Resource." Health Foods Business: March 1991.

Yang, C. S., et al. "Tea and Cancer." Journal of the National Cancer Institute 85 (13):1038–1049.

Zand, Janet. "Herbal Programs for Women's Health." Health Foods Business: 40–41, January 1991.

Zhao, K. S., Mancini, C., and Doria, G. "Enhancement of Immune Response in Mice by Astragalus Menbranaceus Extracts." Immunopharmacology 20:225–243, 1990.

Zhu, Xiao-Dong, and Tang, Xi Can. "Improvement of Impaired Memory in Mice by Huperzine A and Huperzine B." Acta Phamacologica Sinica 6:492–497, 1988.

Zuchrua, Zakay-Rones, Mumcuoglu, M., et al. "Inhibition of Several Strains of Influenza Virus in Vitro and Reduction of Symptoms by an Elderberry Extract (Sambucus nigra) During an Outbreak of Influenza B. Panama." The Journal of Alternative and Complementary Medicine 1:361–369, 1995.

In addition, the following publications have proved to be invaluable resources:

Herbalgram, a newsletter published by the Herb Research Foundation, Austin, Texas.

The Lawrence Review of Natural Products, St. Louis, Missouri.

Pharmacist's Letter, Stockton, California.

Index

....

(Page numbers in **boldface** refer to main entries for specific herbs and problems.)

Now you can achieve optimal health with Dr. Earl Mindell's exclusive formulas!

For the last thirty years, Dr. Mindell has researched and studied the nutrients your body needs on a daily basis in order for it to function at its best and maintain optimal health. In addition to his line of books, Dr. Mindell has created an exclusive line of customized nutritional products based on his latest research. Dr. Mindell's products are not available in stores, so for more information call, write, or fax:

Dr. Earl Mindell
P.O. Box 5400
Milford, CT 06460
1-800-359-3620 (phone)
1-203-882-7255 (fax)

Also enjoy Dr. Earl Mindell's other Fireside guides to healthy living:

Earl Mindell's Anti-Aging Bible	0-684-84909-7	$13.00
Earl Mindell's Food as Medicine	0-684-84907-0	$13.00
Earl Mindell's Secret Remedies	0-684-84910-0	$12.00
Earl Mindell's Soy Miracle	0-684-84908-9	$12.00
Earl Mindell's Soy Miracle Cookbook	0-684-82607-0	$6.95
Earl Mindell's Supplement Bible	0-684-84476-1	$12.00

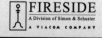